Spiritual Issues and Choices in Dentistry

Edited by
William C. Forbes, D.D.S., M.Div.
Richard G. Topazian, D.D.S.

Christian Medical & Dental Associations
Changing Hearts in Healthcare

The Christian Medical & Dental Associations

The Christian Medical and Dental Associations (CMDA) include the Christian Medical Association (CMA)—physicians and allied medical health-care professionals—and the Christian Dental Association (CDA)—dentists and allied dental healthcare professionals. The combined organization had nearly 14,500 members as of mid-2000.

Prior to May 2000, CMDA was known as the Christian Medical & Dental Society, an organization that was founded in 1931 as the Christian Medical Society. Although the ministry's name has changed to reflect its broadening focus, including a desire to increase its ministry to and with dentists, dental students and allied dental professionals, CMDA's mission remains the same To change the face of healthcare by changing the hearts of doctors.

CMDA provides a variety of ministries to healthcare professionals, including student ministries, marriage growth conferences, short-term domestic and foreign missionary opportunities, medical ethics statements and personal mentoring. For more information, call (423) 844-1000; write CMDA, P.O. Box 7500, Bristol, TN 37621-7500; e-mail: main@cmdahome.org; or, consult the organization's Web site: http://www.cmdahome.org.

The opinions expressed in this book are those of the authors, and may not represent the official position of CMDA on a particular subject.

Advice offered by any author should be viewed as a general guide for the reader's prayerful consideration in the process of his or her personal decision making, in conjunction with input from other trusted sources.

Case studies, illustrations or examples, even when based on the experience or observations of an author, are disguised and/or composites, and not intended to represent any particular person or persons, living or dead.

Unless otherwise identified, all Scripture quotations are taken from the *HOLY BIBLE: NEW INTERNATIONAL VERSION*® (NIV®) COPYRIGHT ©1973, 1978, 1984 by the International Bible Society. Used by permission of Zondervan Publishing House. All rights reserved.

Contents

A WORD FROM THE EDITORS

If you are not a believer in Jesus Christ, we would ask you to read this book anyway and do so with an open mind.

As doctors, our education in science has led some to think that there is no God, or that He is unknowable. Many of us who have examined the evidence, however, hold that belief in God and in his Son, Jesus Christ, is reasonable, rational and intellectually valid. We urge you to consider the evidence anew.

Doubts about God are common, but God himself has promised that those who sincerely seek Him will find Him. The last chapter of this book deals with having a personal relationship with the God of the Universe.

To those readers who do know God, we trust this book will challenge and assist you to deepen your spiritual life, your professional life and your personal life so that you may be more effective for Him in this world.

Thanks. Bill Forbes and Richard Topazian

CHAPTER FOUR

How and Where to Practice

Collin B. Sanford, D.M.D.

Establishment of your practice style and location may seem like a topic best tackled as you end your studious years in dental school. Actually, it's useful to begin thinking of these issues no matter how new you are to the study of dentistry.

Your personality and the factors that have shaped it will also influence the style and location of your future practice. Your style, or manner of treating patients, performing procedures, handling billing, and so forth reveals the kind of person you are—friendly? aloof? meticulous? professional? Your location has to do with where you set up an office, what neighborhoods have access to you, the climate, church, leisure and educational opportunities you require.

With the Lord's help, we can make these all-important decisions and become the best dental professionals possible.

Establishment of your practice style and location may seem like a topic best tackled as you end your studious years in dental school. Actually, the process of making decisions regarding these issues began back when you were considerably younger. The same thought processes are used to decide where and how to practice as those you used to decide where to go to college and where to go to dental school. It's useful to begin thinking of these things no matter how new you are to the study of dentistry. These are decisions that you can shape and mold as you learn more about setting up a practice and determine your preferences over time.

As you proceed through dental school, you will find that there are areas of generalization or specialization which pique your interest.

As you proceed through dental school, you will find that there are areas of generalization or specialization which pique your interest. You may find that academics is your "cup of tea," or that administration is your strong suit. You may respond particularly well to the specialty of a mentor, an admired relative or family friend, and he or she may strongly influence your direction. Your preference may also spring from God-given talent in a particular area which opens doors for you.

Be open to all possibilities and be alert to opportunities as they avail themselves to you. Don't shut the door on anything until you are sure that the opportunity is not for you. Seek God's help in your decision-making processes and He will see you through them.

You have a variety of options once your dental education is complete. Most of us think of practice as the only thing to do, and the majority choose it. But there are other alternatives as well, and some of these alternatives can be meshed together. Academic dentistry is one; administration is another.

In the following pages I will explain and explore the various options so you can begin thinking about where to aim your abilities in order to be most effective professionally and personally. The options in which to practice dentistry can be divided into five major areas: solo practices, partnerships, large groups, academic and administrative dentistry. There are advantages and disadvantages to each.

Dentistry Options
Solo Practice

Solo practice has many benefits. If you decide to become a solo practitioner, which the majority of practitioners in the United States are, you can control how you practice, whom you hire, how many hours you want to work and what those hours are. You decide which areas of specialty you will perform in the office and which you will refer to other practitioners. You can choose whether to profit-share with your staff or assume all profits of the company yourself. Other than state and federal regulations, you will answer only to yourself and your patients in all that you do.

Although solo practice is usually very lucrative, it can also be lonely.

Although solo practice is usually very lucrative, it can also be lonely. You have minimal interaction with other professionals on a daily basis. To offset the isolation, you can take continuing education, belong to study groups and go to many of the professional meetings. You may find that you are the kind of individual who thrives in such an environment.

Other downsides to solo practice besides isolation include difficulty in getting away from the office, even briefly. Since you have no one to cover for you, people will depend on you alone for their dental needs and emergencies. Even though you sometimes need time away to relax and think about something besides dentistry, you may find making arrangements for absences to be problematic. As well, even if you do get time away, the overhead of the office continues, even when you are not there. I practiced by myself for the first eight years of my private practice life, and I found that leaving the office for a ten-day missions trip cost more than just the trip expenses. I also lost approximately $5,000-8,000 a week in revenue, wages and general office overhead. I have no regrets about incurring those losses in order to serve on missionary trips, but I still had to count the cost.

Partnerships

Partnerships in dentistry have enabled many dentists to overcome some of the liabilities of the solo practice environment. Two dentists sharing an office allows for daily professional interaction. You can take all of the courses you want, yet you can also discuss problems and treatment plans with a fellow professional. Coverage of the office during vacations and continuing education becomes much easier, as long as you don't take your vacations at the same time.

The downsides to this style of practice include some diminishing independence when you are no longer in charge. You can't make decisions completely on your own when it comes to office management, hiring and firing, hours of operation and purchasing of equipment, among other things. Some offices have clear delineations of the tasks and responsibilities of each partner, but there remain many issues that need to be resolved by both partners. Being in a partnership is like being in a marriage, so it becomes imperative that the individuals involved are very clear regarding their goals, expectations and compatibility. Even though it would seem that there would be more revenue to be generated and more efficiency in the running of a partnership, data shows that dentists actually make less as partners than as solo practitioners.[1]

Large Groups

Large groups take partnerships a step further in the professional interaction aspect of dentistry. In a group office, several individuals are accessible for consultation and interaction, some of whom may be specialists. There is minimal need to refer anyone out of the office for care, since the practice likely can handle the vast majority of the needs of its patients.

Large groups can commonly afford the newest equipment and devices on the market and groups are often more willing to make these kinds of investments.

Large groups can commonly afford the newest equipment and devices on the market and groups are often more willing to make these kinds of investments. Coverage for vacation and other time out of the office can be easily accommodated. Hiring, firing, general office management and details of office protocol are frequently left to an office manager, which allows professionals who perform dentistry to do precisely that, without being overly concerned with administration of the office.

As ideal as this may seem, this option isn't without its problems. Most dentists are individuals who like control, and giving this up to someone else can be difficult. As you get into larger groups, you increasingly lose individual control, and the need to get along with others is premium. Another potential problem in a large group, particularly for a young dentist recently out of school or residency training, is the typically long and expensive period required before one can become a full partner. This time and expense can often be overwhelming to the ambitious young person with a definite time line. On the other hand, this type of practice can be ideal for an individual who wants to practice part-time or who really wants to do only clinical dentistry, take home a salary and have minimal practice responsibilities.

Academic Dentistry

Academic dentistry may afford you the opportunity to practice part-time, should you desire to do so. It also offers other opportunities which are not available to you as a practitioner. For many dentists, the desire to do research is strong, and, in most cases, only the academic world can afford you this opportunity. There are other ways to get involved with research, but the networking and educational resources within a dental school are very difficult to match outside the university environment. A university provides professionals the opportunity to teach students, residents and graduate students. To many, this allure is great, and the education environment can be very stimulating and gratifying. Professional interaction is probably at its highest level in this type of environment. There are generally set times when you are at the university (being on call is rare); vacation and free time can be taken without fear that the university, unlike a practice, will shut down without your presence.

For many dentists, the desire to do research is strong, and, in most cases, only the academic world can afford you this opportunity.

The downsides to academic dentistry may not be a problem for every dentist. In academia, you are not your own boss—there is always someone above you to whom you must answer. This may be a department chair, a dean, a provost, vice president of a university or even a state political system. This is not necessarily bad, and can even prove beneficial to your career. Often these people can provide leadership and guidance for you in your academic pursuits. You may not be able to take your vacation when you desire, since you're tied to teaching schedules, lab commitments or filling in for another instructor. In these instances, more than just the patients you would have had in practice will demand your time—

Combinations of the various dental options have also proven to be very satisfying.

courses, meetings, students, preparation for teaching and research endeavors which allow you to work toward promotion and tenure will take hours from your days.

One note of caution about academics: If this is an area you seriously want to pursue, I encourage you to speak to someone who has done it well and successfully. Obtain his or her wisdom regarding the additional education, advanced degrees and research training needed to be an effective faculty member.

Administrative Dentistry

As I mentioned earlier, administration in dentistry is a growing field of opportunity, especially in the areas of governmental oversight and insurance industry intervention. As much as most of us don't want to think about these issues, they are real and they will not be going away in the near future. Dentists must be involved in the administration of these programs in order to ensure that the patients receive the best possible care. Treatment decisions should be made by individuals who know dentistry, rather than by pure administrators who have minimal working knowledge of the profession. Often, an additional business degree or a public health degree will be necessary to function in these areas.

The advantages of this type of career somewhat reflect those of the academic side of dentistry—fringe benefits, vacation time, freedom to be away from the office, etc. In addition, this type of career provides opportunities for those dentists who may be disabled or who have decided they do not want to do clinical dentistry.

The disadvantages are also similar to the academic career in that you must always answer to someone. In addition, you may have to deal with unhappy dentists who feel that decisions made by a third party are unfair for their patients.

Combinations of the different options listed have also proven to be very satisfying. Combining private practice's positive features with those of administrative dentistry can provide a career of great challenge and fulfillment. I have been fortunate to combine a full-time private practice partnership with a part-time (two half-days per week) faculty position at a university. This combination has been ideal for me and my family's needs.

Dentistry Style

Once you are settled into the professional environment you have chosen, your sense of style will come into play. As I said before, it's never too early to start thinking about this area. As you ponder your options, consider these questions:

- Do you interact with people more formally or casually?
- Do you want people to call you "Doctor" all of the time, only in the office, only in front of certain patients, peers . . . or never?
- Will you call all of your patients by their first names, or will you be selective about with whom you are more formal?
- Will you dress formally (suit or tie) for work every day?
- What will you expect from your staff in terms of formality with patients and with you?
- What message will the office decor relay?
- Will you be compatible with and happy with a staff person who is very informal in his or her approach if you are at the other extreme of formality?

How you interact with both your staff and your patients will ultimately influence how you practice and how happy you are.

These questions may seem somewhat superficial, yet they do become important. How you interact with both your staff and your patients will ultimately influence how you practice and how happy you are. Starting my career in academic dentistry forced me to be much more formal than I wanted to be. Private practice has allowed me to decide for myself the style of my office. I have been able to choose the equipment, supplies, laboratories, types of dentistry I want to refer out, office decor and staffing patterns I prefer.

Although most of us work out the answers to these questions over time, they are areas to consider that will help you avoid some of the pitfalls when entering practice. I found that I made many mistakes when entering practice because I did not take the opportunity to think through most of these issues. I was fortunate that I was older—thirty-three—when I entered the private practice arena, thus perhaps more secure than some in my abilities and personality. Still, my lack of forethought forced me to reverse field often.

I was shortsighted regarding sizes and types of office supplies, the kind of copy machine we really needed, the fact that a computer was essential, the amount of part-time help required and most importantly, the actual size of the office.

Practice Location

Determining where you will practice your profession can be an overwhelming task. There are many factors that come into play as you make this decision. Some of these factors you have reasonable control over, and others are out of your control. Should you decide to do specialty training, residency training or to go into academia, for example, acceptance to these programs is out of your control. Sometimes you can choose the location of your dental school and your postgraduate education; these are often important issues in determining where you may want to practice. They also provide opportunities for you to find associateships or academic possibilities. Contacts within these environments can be excellent sources of information and opportunities.

There are many factors that come into play as you make the decision of where to practice.

Determining where you want to be for the remainder of your life is a multifaceted decision. One should bear in mind the fact that very few of us will stay in one location, or even in one vocation, for the remainder of our lives. Most likely we will have several locations, and spouse and family will often play a major role in this decision. Other factors which may influence your decision include academic and teaching opportunities, location (urban, suburban or rural), climate and church affiliation.

Spouse/Family

If you are married or anticipate becoming married, your spouse will have a great impact on this decision. It is imperative that both of you are happy and satisfied with your location. If not, it can create problems within your family life that are not easily resolved.

I heard about a colleague who completed dental school and opened a very successful practice in her home town. She became financially secure. However, her spouse was extremely unhappy in the climate where the practice was located. After twenty years of frustration in the home, the family moved to a climate where both individuals could be happy. Had my colleague chosen with her spouse's preferences in mind initially, they could have avoided the strife they endured for so long and the move they eventually had to make.

Take your spouse's feelings and desires into account. As well, consider how close you want to live to extended family and how easily different family members can travel, should you live long distances apart.

Choosing the style and location of practice that best suits you and those you love must be approached with common sense, a thorough knowledge of what you are getting yourself into, and prayer.

Academic/Teaching Opportunities

Obviously, if you remain in academics, you will need to be in an environment which allows you to pursue your academic interest. Finding a location to do this may have more to do with what is available to you than what you personally desire. There are certainly opportunities available in many places throughout the country, and even abroad. Criteria by which to evaluate each site rests with you, but thorough knowledge of promotion and tenure requirements is essential. Seek out the advice of individuals who have a working knowledge of what the expectations will be for you to be successful as an academic dentist.

There may be opportunities to teach, even if you choose not to pursue a purely academic career. Many dental schools utilize private practitioners to do clinical teaching, as do many residency training programs.

(Consider, as well, the future educational needs of the family you have, or plan to have, in making your decision.) A key factor in your decision-making process is how much contact you desire/require with professional associates. And remember: Academics often require moves for promotion.

Location

Where will you be happiest practicing your profession? One of dentistry's most attractive qualities is that dentists can practice virtually wherever they desire; this is not possible in most vocations. There are advantages and disadvantages in urban, suburban and rural locations.

One of dentistry's most attractive qualities is that dentists can practice virtually wherever they desire.

If you practice in an urban environment, many of your patients will be individuals who work in the city. You may not treat their families. The individuals who live near your practice and come to you for care will differ greatly depending on the city in which you practice. A rural practice will offer the opposite scenario: lots of family practice.

First of all, decide how far you are willing to travel to work. Do you want to live in the suburbs and travel to the city to practice, or live and work in a rural setting? Some find a long drive drudgery, others enjoy the time as an opportunity to "wind down."

Then too, there's your life outside the practice to consider. Will you want to live in an urban environment with its advantages of social and cultural activities, or will you prefer instead to live with fewer crowds and more quiet?

Are the suburbs a good option for you? If you practice in the suburbs or rurally, it is likely you will see more families, and you will be more involved in the lives of your patients, both in and out of the office. Does that suit you?

Climate

I have already mentioned the issue of the climate in which you wish to settle. It is a multifaceted decision. What type of climate will make you and your family happy for the majority of the year? Do you desire one temperature all year long, or do you enjoy the changing seasons? Do the leisure activities you enjoy require warm or cold weather or both? How far are you willing to travel to reach the leisure activities that you desire? If you are a windsurfer and love the ocean, do not practice in North Dakota. On the other hand, if you are an avid skier, it may not make sense to live in Florida. This is not to say that you can't travel to participate in these activities, but living close to them is much more convenient.

Church Affiliation

What church requirements are essential to you? Do you feel a need to be involved with a large church or a small one? Do you want a church with an active youth program or one that ministers to single adults? Wherever you practice, there will be churches that can meet your individual and family needs.

Involvement in a church is very rewarding and fulfilling, and I would encourage you to visit churches in the area in which you are planning to settle. This will give you a feel for the community, its environment and commitment; it will also give you a feel for the people who worship there.

Having the support of a church family can be very beneficial to you, not only if you are settling in a new community, but also if you have been in the community for a long time. My wife and I both appreciate the fact that our church is where we spend most of our leisure time. Our church has become a second family to us, and we would find separation from this very traumatic should we ever have to move.

Your Decision

Ultimately, you must decide what style of practice and location of practice best suit you and those you love. You must approach theses issues with common sense, a thorough knowledge of what you are getting yourself into . . . and prayer. Take your time in researching your various options. If a certain type of professional life appeals to you, by all means, visit someone who is doing it. Get a good, honest look at the way of life you think you want.

The Bible says in Proverbs to trust in the Lord "with all your heart." By so doing, you will find the style and location choices easier to evaluate. As you work in tandem with the Lord, He will guide you through the decisions and give you the wisdom and courage to make them, so you can be the best possible dental professional He envisions.

Notes

1. P. E. Anderson, "Dentists respond to Annual Practice Survey," *Dental Economics* 87 (1986): 30-48.

CHAPTER FIVE

Principles of Ethical Decision Making

Being morally virtuous asks us to apply the basics of ethical practice to all aspects of our lives, including family life. What we are at home, we also must be in our professional lives.

Fred C. Bergamo, D.D.S.

Consider the following scenarios. In each case, what would you do?

> *The crown that I am fitting on tooth #28 seats pretty well, but not quite all the way. The margin is open on the lingual, but the cement should fill that in, for a number of years anyway. Who will know the difference? And why put the patient through the inconvenience of doing a remake? Of course, I could blame it on the lab, but when I figure in the extra-time cost that eats away at my profit. . . .*

◆

To handle such situations with wisdom requires a firm ethical foundation.

After two Carpules of lidocaine, and forty-five minutes of chair time, the huge occlusal prep in tooth #31 was complete. With a little nudge of the bur towards the distal, we could make this a DO and recoup some money lost due to the extra time it took to restore this tooth. After all, we are already taking a loss on this procedure because the patient has "managed care" insurance, and we'll be getting 41 percent less than our usual fee. That extra twenty dollars would help ease our "pain."

♦

Mary Hygienist completed the scaling and root planing, finished up with a rophy and preliminary charting for cavities and defective restorations, and called Dr. Jones for the exam. Mary was convinced that all existing restorations were in acceptable condition. Dr. Jones immediately diagnosed the need for crowns on teeth #3, 5, and 15. Mary was stunned! Just six months earlier, Dr. Jones never would have made this diagnosis. The existing restorations were in perfect condition. What were his motives? Were the building of his opulent new home and the associated financial pressures affecting his treatment planning? Maybe that's why he'd been snapping at the staff for no good reason. The office mood was changing, and suddenly, so were the diagnoses. . . .

♦

The Farnham family were always stretching "patient rights" to the limit. They had figured out long ago that old Doc Alloy could be taken advantage of. Their response to his generosity included broken appointments, broken promises to meet financial arrangements made in good faith, even some unkind comments around the community when the Doc did draw a line in the sand and demand payment of a long-overdue balance. Dr. Alloy's young associate, Dr. Marks, does not agree with his superior on this issue, and many heated debates occur. Dr. Marks argues for "principles," for running an efficient, well-managed office that eliminates those patients who constantly violate office policy and affect the profit line and office morale. Dr. Alloy argues for patience, for compassion, for going the extra mile. He defends the Farnhams' social circumstances: their kids can't be denied needed dental care just because of their parents' ignorance. In frustration, Dr. Alloy exclaims, "Where are your ethics, Marks? Don't you know there is more to dental practice than just the bottom line?" To which the young doctor replies, "If we allow our bottom line to be trashed by undisciplined patients, we will have no decent practice in which to showcase our ethics."

Discussion:

All dentists face similar points of decision every day. However, each dentist's reaction can become highly subjective. In the above, would your responses be the same as mine? Should they be? With the multitude of dental personalities and practice situations that exist, can we expect unanimous agreement regarding what to do with the crown on tooth #28, the billing for tooth #31, the diagnosis for teeth #3, 5, and 15, and the case of the Farnham family? Does a single right decision exist? Setting unanimity aside, we are still left with the individual dentist, *you*—how will you decide? What will guide you in making a decision?

Throughout the ages we have been given varied and useful sources upon which to develop our ethical standards.

To handle such situations with wisdom requires a firm ethical foundation. Simply stated, *ethics* concerns our moral dealings in every area of life, personal and professional. The terms "morals" and "ethics" are often used interchangeably, and though they are related, they are not the same. *Morals* describes what is usual or customary for a society, the behavior and relationships of its people, and "how they ought to behave towards one another in order to live in peace and harmony." Ethics refers to the disciplined, systematic, reasoned theory that might support specific moral judgments. Ethics is the systematic reflection of morals.[1]

Sources of Ethics

Throughout the ages we have been given varied and useful sources upon which to develop our ethical standards. Many cultures have passed on to us their concepts of "rights" and "wrongs." The ancient philosopher Plato suggested that there are at least four universal ideas of basic virtue: courage, temperance, wisdom and justice. Subsequent thinkers have presented a number of approaches to ethical decision making, three of which we will consider in the context of this chapter. (Because of space constraints, we will survey these only briefly. Please see the bibliography for sources that discuss these ideas in detail.)

The school of philosophy that appeals to natural law asserts that all normal human beings share certain basic moral rights and instincts. The apostle Paul alludes to this basic moral code that is written on man's heart and conscience in Romans 1 and 2. Even though consensus is often hard to achieve in our society, our customs and traditions still stimulate a concern for the basic welfare of human beings. Providing for the general welfare has worthy examples in the humanitarian and spiritual ministries of organizations such as the Salvation Army, World Vision and the scores of rescue missions found in the major cities of the world.

Even though consensus is often hard to achieve in our society, our customs and traditions still stimulate a concern for the basic welfare of human beings.

Another moral tradition founds itself on the concept of utilitarianism, i.e., the concern that the greatest good is done for the greatest number of individuals. What is critical are the consequences of our decisions and actions, and these are right if they do more good than any alternative action.

A third approach—deontology (the study of moral obligation)—approaches this from a different direction. A deontologist maintains that what is right and good is not always that which produces the most good for the most people. Keeping promises, honesty, truth telling, autonomy and justice, when applied specifically, do not necessarily affect the larger group positively. The deontologist's moral obligations do not depend entirely on the value (good or bad) of the consequences his actions cause. He is concerned with doing good, but his actions will be governed by a set of virtues that will take priority over the outcome of his action.

For the Christian seriously exploring the realm of ethics, the Scriptures provide the ultimate source of guidance. The apostle Paul, writing to Timothy, stated that "All Scripture is God-breathed and is useful for teaching, rebuking, correcting and training in righteousness, so that the man of God may be thoroughly equipped for every good work" (2 Timothy 3:16-17). The Ten Commandments provide us with the eternal standard of God's righteousness. God, through Moses, presented commandments (not suggestions) that strictly regulated man's relationship with his neighbor and with God. Centuries later, the prophet Micah, crying out for social justice, delivered God's message to sinful Israel. In response to Israel's offer to give sacrifices for her sins, Micah declares God's preference: "He has showed you, O man, what is good. And what does the Lord require of you? To act justly and to love mercy and to walk humbly with your God" (Micah 6:8).

For the Christian seriously exploring the realm of ethics, the Scriptures provide the ultimate source of guidance.

As well, there are other, more specific laws the Christian dentist can look to for guidance. Historically, civil authority was probably the earliest regulator of medical practice. In the Babylonian Laws of Hammurabi (2200 B.C.) eight of the 282 sections dealt with the fee scales of physicians. With regard to the oral cavity, the Law offers the directive: "If a man has made the tooth of a man that is his equal fall out, one shall make *his* tooth fall out. If he has made the tooth of a poor man fall out he should pay 1/3 of a mina of silver."[2] (Italics mine.)

The earliest known professional code is the Hippocratic Oath (500 B.C.). It embodied four main principles: 1) Advance the profession rather than the individual doctor; 2) never use medical knowledge to injure but always to help the patient; 3) defer to specialist assistance whatever is in the best interest of the patient; 4) maintain professional secrecy.

In 1866, the American Dental Association (ADA) adopted its first Code of Ethics, which has been continually refined and expanded over the years. The ADA Principles of Ethics and Code of Professional Conduct provide us with a public standard by which to judge ourselves and our profession. They are constantly revised to address the issues currently confronting us as dentists. As well, a strong movement has developed within the profession to bring the study of ethics to the forefront. Many dental schools now include a course in ethics in the core curriculum. Students are guided through case histories, asked to weigh the principles of right and wrong and challenged to systematically determine a right course of action.

The renewed interest in professional ethics also spawned the formation of Professional Ethics in Dentistry Network (PEDNET), an international group of dentists and non-dentists interested in the education of professional ethics in dentistry. It sponsors seminars that deal with issues such as advertising, third-party relationships, research integrity, OSHA, doctor/patient relationships and mediation. Its members actively publish articles on ethical issues and offer moral and ethical perspectives on major policy and practice issues.

There is no law which prevents you or me from offering a patient two restorative choices, neglecting to disclose a less costly third alternative.

Still, while civil authority continues to regulate the practice of dentistry and medicine, we have never outgrown Hippocrates' maxims, and though the dental profession itself seeks to regulate its practitioners' moral behavior, none can control the conscience of the individual and his or her response to ethical challenges. Even laws, authorities and maxims have limitations.

For example, one's conduct may be unethical and still legal. There is no law which prevents you or me from offering a patient two restorative choices, neglecting to disclose a less costly third alternative. Thus we need more than rules; we need determination to follow those directives.

Principles for Decision Making

As one reflects on the various sources discussed that have impacted dental ethics, it becomes obvious that professional behavior can reflect all of the above. Just what the behavioral mix will be depends upon the individual. Is he or she dogmatic, conservative and rigid? Or perhaps, is he or she very liberal, flexible and compromising? Or even a combination of these? The rigors of daily practice confront us with ethical problems that force us to ask some hard questions: What ought I to do? What difference will it make? Who will know the difference—and does that matter? How will my ethics be judged in the light of this action?

Certain basic principles or virtues can act as guides to ethical living. The Harvard ethicist Arthur Dyck has formulated a list of ethical principles that provides a valuable resource for consideration when we are faced with a dilemma.

They are:

1. Promise keeping: trust, confidentiality.
2. Truth telling: honesty, sincerity.
3. Reparation: making up for a wrong.
4. Gratitude: appreciation.
5. Justice: fair and equal treatment.
6. Beneficence: doing good.
7. Non-maleficence: avoiding doing harm.
8. Being morally virtuous.[3]

Certain basic principles or virtues can act as guides to ethical living.

We can derive a number of general applications from these.

1. Promise keeping: Trust and Confidentiality

The relationship between dentist and patient is essentially one of unequals. The patient is in a vulnerable position. He must trust the dentist to deliver the level of care which is within the bounds of good dental practice. By accepting that patient into his or her practice, the dentist makes a commitment to deliver dental care to the best of his or her ability, and to follow through with any promises made to the patient regarding type and quality of dental care. Compassionate care must be coupled with a commitment to professional confidentiality. The dentist has an ethical responsibility to refrain from abusing his or her position of power. Respect and trust for each other is the norm for a healthy doctor/patient relationship.

2. Truth telling: Honesty and Sincerity

The patient and the dentist both have the right to clear and truthful communication. The patient has the obligation to provide an accurate health history. The dentist is obliged to provide an accurate and truthful diagnosis of the patient's dental health. Dishonesty on the part of either one can lead to dangerous compromises in therapy.

3. Reparation: Making Up for a Wrong

What we are at home, we also must be in our professional lives.

The ethical dentist has the obligation to "make things right." At times the best treatment plans fail. Or, for example, not every impression is perfect on the first take. Sometimes the marginal ridge of the freshly packed amalgam breaks off when the band is removed. Is the patient always aware of these mistakes? Perhaps not. But the dentist has the ethical obligation to remake or retake and to ensure the proper result. The same is true of major "mistakes."

4. Gratitude: Appreciation

Most dentists consider this an attitude that the *patient* should have. After all, patients come for the alleviation or prevention of pain, for cosmetic renovation and general oral health services. The successful dentist should be the recipient of the patient's gratitude. On the other hand, the dentist must be grateful for the patient's trust of his or her technical skill and professional judgment. The dentist is also aware that the patient helps support his or her standard of living, and this enters into the doctor's attitude of gratitude as well.

5. Justice: Fair and Equal Treatment

This principle provides a tremendous challenge to the dental healthcare system. How can dental services be fair and equal when patients come with differing needs and financial resources? To equalize the availability of dental care in the local population seems unreasonable. And yet, the ethical local dentist, motivated to do justice, can make a difference. Not all patients have equal available funds, but they can all be treated with the same level of compassion and care. The dentist can adjust his or her fee scale at times to help the family with legitimate financial problems. Volunteering dental services through the state or local dental societies can assist those who are truly needy.

6. Beneficence: Doing Good

The imperative to do good, to be good, to work and serve for the good of mankind is with us from childhood. This is the foundation for servanthood, the core of the Golden Rule: "Do unto others as you would have them do unto you."

Sometimes patients reject our efforts to do good. They may request a lesser "good," which we view as "harm." Still, the imperative to do good is inescapable. Our professional codes demand it; our personal standards require it; our community expects it.

7. Non-maleficence: Not Doing Harm

This principle is the cornerstone of the Latin phrase: "*Primum, Non Nocere*—First of all, do no harm." This ethic seeks to dissuade any clinician from professional bungling and technical risk-taking. The dentist must always be cognizant of his or her technical limitations, avoiding venturing into areas of practice for which he or she is not trained, or in which he or she lacks competence. The doctor must avoid the pressure of the patient who says, "You can do it, Doc. You're good at everything else." By the same token, routine procedures should not receive casual attention to the extent that they become sloppy and substandard dentistry thus becomes possible.

Ethical problems, when they do arise, are better handled when a high moral standard is the norm for a practice.

8. Being Morally Virtuous

Dyck puts the ultimate challenge on the table. Unless one has this reality in place in his or her life, fulfilling the previous principles becomes an even greater challenge. A personal ethic cannot simply be carried on a card in one's wallet with the hope that it will somehow leak out and affect how one lives and practices dentistry. Being morally virtuous asks us to apply the basics of ethical practice to all aspects of our lives, including family life. What we are at home, we also must be in our professional lives.

A Systematic Approach

Arthur Dyck's list of ethical principles provides a practical source with which the concerned dentist can begin to examine his or her professional ethics and behavior. To apply those principles in specific occasions of decision making, it is useful to consider a format suggested by the revered German theologian and martyr to the Third Reich, Dietrich Bonhoeffer. In his work, *Ethics,* Bonhoeffer offers a five-point plan for the responsible man or woman to follow: "It is he himself who must observe, judge, weigh up, decide and act."[4]

Applying this fivefold challenge to our daily practice, we are asked to:

Observe: Examine, gather pertinent information and the necessary diagnostic aids with which to reach a decision.

Judge: Examine and separate the relevant from the irrelevant.

Weigh Up: Reflect upon, ponder the ethical implications presented by the case; examine conscience, personal values, professional codes of ethics and scriptural truths.

Decide: Take a position and stand by it.

Act: Move upon the conclusions of our decision-making process and live with the consequences.

This systematic approach to ethical problems in dental practice should enable the doctor to make wise decisions and avoid problems of misunderstanding, conflicts of interest and even malpractice.

Above All . . . Love

The Christian dentist must excel in love for his or her neighbors, patients and staff. The doctor's practice should be known for its compassion, for its ability to treat each patient as that stranger to whom Jesus refers in Matthew 25:34-40 as the "least of these brothers of mine."

The practice must deliver dental care to the dentist's fellow man or woman as if it were for Christ Himself. Kindness and a caring attitude are all too often swept aside by the drive for efficiency in the modern dental practice. Ethical problems, when they do arise, are better handled when a high moral standard is the norm for a practice. To this must be added a commitment to a high technical standard. Careless, substandard dentistry has no place in a self-proclaimed ethical practice. This can lead to undue stress, which is common in many dental practices and provides fertile ground for errors in judgment and behavior.

In light of all these principles and guidelines, I suggest that you revisit and reconsider the difficult scenarios listed at the beginning of the chapter, asking yourself how an ethical dentist might resolve each case.

The Christian dentist's practice must deliver dental care to his fellow man or woman as of it were to Christ Himself.

Conclusion:

Codes, laws, maxims and scriptural commands may all contribute to the guidance of the dentist who actively seeks to practice ethically. The Christian dentist may consider each of these, while also recognizing the need to interpret the circumstances of a particular problem with a mind renewed by the Holy Spirit and motivated by love.

In the area of decision making, human reason is essential, but for the Christian, reason cannot operate independently of God's particular guidance.

Our Lord offers not just an ethic of love—"Love your neighbor as yourself" (Matthew 22:39)—but He enters the lives of all who receive Him and He supplies the dynamic that can empower that ethic. This adds up to justice, honesty, forgiveness, gratitude, promise keeping, beneficence, virtue and then some.

The New Testament further associates Jesus with humility and compassion, while asserting that we are to be like Him if we claim Him as Savior.

If we claim to be Christians ("Christ's ones"), our patients should be able to detect a difference in the way we conduct dental practice. Hopefully they will be able to see not just strong, reliable ethics, but Christ in us showing His love to them through us.

Notes

1. James T. Rule and Robert M. Veatch, *Ethical Questions in Dentistry* (Carol Stream, IL: Quintessence Books, 1993), p. 40.
2. "The History of Medicine and Surgery," *Encyclopedia Britannica,* Vol. 23, pp.885-889.
3. Arthur J. Dyck, *On Human Care: An Introduction to Ethics* (Nashville: Abingdon, 1977), p. 160.
4. Dietrich Bonhoeffer, *Ethics*, ed. Eberhard Bethge, trans. Neville Horton Smith (New York: Macmillan, 1962), p. 217.

Bibliography

Bergamo, Fred C., and Lewis P. Bird. *A Personal Probe: Ethical Problems In Dental Practice.* Bristol, TN: Christian Medical & Dental Society, 1980.

Carnahan, Charles. *The Dentist and the Law.* St. Louis: Mosby, 1955.

Davis, John Jefferson. *Evangelical Ethics.* Phillipsburg, NJ: Presbyterian and Reformed Publishing Company, 1985.

Edmunds, V., and C. G. Scorer. *Medical Ethics: A Christian View.* London: Tyndale Press, 1958.

Geisler, Norman L. *Christian Ethics: Options and Issues.* Grand Rapids: Baker Book House, 1995.

Harron, F., J. Burnside, and T. Beauchamp. *Health and Human Values.* New Haven, CT: Yale University Press, 1983.

Henry, Carl F. H. *Baker's Dictionary of Christian Ethics.* Grand Rapids: Baker Book House, 1973.

Mott, Stephen C. *Biblical Ethics and Social Change.* New York: Oxford University Press, 1982.

Ozar, David T., and David Sokol. *Dental Ethics at Chairside.* St. Louis: Mosby, 1995.

Reeck, Darrell. *Ethics for the Professions, A Christian Perspective.* Minneapolis: Augsburg Publishing House 1982.

Ryrie, Charles C. *Biblical Answers to Contemporary Issues.* Chicago: Moody Bible Institute, 1991.

Stott, John. *Decisive Issues Facing Christians Today.* Grand Rapids: Baker Book House, 1990.

Warner, R., and H. Segal. *Ethical Issues of Informed Consent in Dentistry.* Chicago: Quintessence Publishing Company, 1980.

CHAPTER SIX

The Biblical Rationale for Service to the Poor

Nowadays, even routine and preventive dental care can be very expensive. Who will be the Good Samaritan for the working poor and their families?

William C. Forbes, D.D.S., M.Div.

Christian dentists are in a unique position to relieve the suffering of the poor, not just in some far-off country, but wherever they work. Every practice has a population of disadvantaged and disenfranchised people in the area, and many more exist outside those boundaries as well. How we deal with this ubiquitous situation reflects our response to a large part of the Scriptures, for the Bible often speaks of our responsibility to the poor.

Let us consider first the extent of the need.

The Need

The Christian Medical and Dental Associations' ethical statement on *Health Care for the Poor* says:

> "The . . . burgeoning price tag for health care is transforming medicine from its position as a humanitarian outreach to one in which it is seen by many as a runaway dollar-consumer that needs to be reined in. Many of the recent changes in the business side of medicine, e.g. DRGs, HMOs, and changes in the provisions of Medicare and Medicaid have been made primarily for reasons of cost containment. Unfortunately, no method aimed principally at saving money has yet been put into effect that has not somehow rationed care based on a patient's ability to pay at least part of the bill. The corollary of this is that comprehensive health care is increasingly available to those who can afford it, but increasingly unavailable to those who cannot."[1]

There are those who desire good dental care for their families, but simply cannot afford to pay the bill.

There are many patients who are not poor enough to qualify for government assistance, but who are too poor to pay dental bills. These are the working poor, who desire good dental care for their families, but simply cannot afford to pay the bill. In my practice, a family of five, which had two routine six-month checkups and, say, sealants and three moderate restorations in the course of a year, faced a yearly dental bill somewhere in the range of $1,000. This is without root-canal therapy, partials or crowns.

Regardless of the fact that these types of treatments are a good investment, health-wise, for any family, such expenses simply will not fit into the budget of the working poor.

Charitable organizations providing health care for the poor in the United States have addressed this need in a number of different ways. Historically, dental clinics were set up in hospitals and other healthcare facilities for treatment of indigent dental patients. There, volunteer and salaried dentists and hygienists treated patients. But in recent years, many places have abandoned that model, and are increasingly serving only as screening and referral facilities. People are then sent to dentists who have agreed in advance to see them under a variety of guidelines. These guidelines vary from dentist to dentist. One dentist may set aside a day a month or a morning a month to see patients referred from the screening facility. Another dentist may work the needy person in with regular patients, but set a limit on the number of people seen each month. Each dentist establishes his or her own parameters, and the referral agency works within those parameters.

There was a time when dental care was not as expensive as it is now. Dental care wasn't as good then, either.

The referral system has advantages: dentists usually are more comfortable working in their own offices, with familiar equipment and staff, and clinics do not have to deal with increased costs of maintaining and supplying their own facilities.

As well as the referral system works, though, the unfortunate fact remains that most areas of the country remain greatly underserved. Severe shortages have been encountered by many clinics. These clinics may have a fully-equipped dental operatory, but only one dentist who will volunteer one day a month, to see about seven patients. Some clinics have tried to acquire services of dental students, but have problems getting dentists to supervise those students. They have tried to get help from retired dentists, but have been unsuccessful. They may have a young dentist in the area who will take Medicare and Medicaid patients. Some of the patients may go to a dental school clinic, but these opportunities are severely limited.

There was a time when dental care was not as expensive as it is now. Dental care wasn't as good then, either. But in those days, working people could pay their own dental bills as long as they did not have major problems. Nowadays, even routine and preventive care can be very expensive, and restorative treatments can run to thousands of dollars for a single tooth. Obviously, there is a problem with access to dental care. Who will be the Good Samaritan for these working poor and their families?

The Biblical Rationale

Could it be that we are actually treating the Lord Jesus Christ when we treat a needy patient? Do we see it as a chance to ease the pain of our Lord Himself?

There is no question that our Lord considered charity toward the poor a very high priority for the Christian. In Matthew 25, Jesus describes the actions that separated true believers in Christ from false ones:

> "I was hungry and you gave me something to eat, I was thirsty and you gave me something to drink, I was a stranger and you invited me in, I needed clothes and you clothed me, I was sick and you looked after me, I was in prison and you came to visit me" (Matthew 25:35-36).

When the believers can't recall performing these services for the Lord [the King] Himself, He tells them, "Whatever you did for one of the least of these brothers of mine, you did for me" (verse 40).

Could it be that we are actually treating the Lord Jesus Christ when we treat a needy patient? Do we see it as a chance to ease the pain of our Lord Himself? Or do we see simply a person who is too ignorant to take care of his teeth, too lazy to get a job so he could pay us, too inconsiderate to say "thank you," too dishonest to admit that he doesn't even intend to pay the bill?

Such attitudes don't mesh with Scriptures such as Hebrews 13:1-2:

> "Keep on loving each other as brothers. Do not forget to entertain strangers, for by so doing some people have entertained angels without knowing it."

Again the Scriptures exhort us to treat strangers as more than they appear to be: even as angels, sometimes . . . but always as people created in the image of God, Himself.

When the practicing dentist treats the disadvantaged, he must never lose sight of the fact that the patient, whether able to pay or not, is a creation of God and deserves to be treated with dignity and respect. As Christians, we cannot allow our service to indigent patients to be "second class." Treating patients in a demeaning way demeans ourselves and our witness for Christ in the community. We do not practice only for the money. We practice to provide a service, and if we provide that service only to the wealthy or those with the ability to pay, we lose sight of what service really is—which is what we are all about.

We are to emulate our Lord, who "did not come to be served, but to serve, and to give his life as a ransom for many" (Matthew 20:28).

After all, do we have any reason to treat anyone as somehow "less" than we ourselves are? When we became Christians, we were justified in God's sight; that is, we were made just as if we had never sinned, and therefore eligible for the blessings of the Christian life. We don't earn such blessings through our faithful obedience, for we would all fail. We are justified by our faith; that much is made clear by the Scriptures.

The rationale, then, for serving the disadvantaged and disenfranchised with charitable dental treatment is obedience to God's Word, which tells us explicitly to serve all in love. We must love all men equally, because that's the way the Lord created us:

We must never lose sight of the fact that our patient, whether able to pay or not, is a creation of God and deserves to be treated with dignity and respect.

> "You have heard that it was said, 'Love your neighbor and hate your enemy.' But I tell you: Love your enemies and pray for those who persecute you, that you may be sons of your Father in heaven" (Matthew 5:43-45).

There are many more Scriptures affirming God's attitude toward the oppressed and poor. I will list only a few:

> "Love your neighbor as yourself" (Matthew 19:19).

> "Give to the one who asks you, and do not turn away from the one who wants to borrow from you" (Matthew 5:42).

Christian dentists and dental students need to keep in mind that their primary calling is to faith in Christ, and dentistry is a secondary calling.

"He who oppresses the poor to increase his wealth and he who gives gifts to the rich—both come to poverty" (Proverbs 22:16).

"He who is kind to the poor lends to the LORD, and he will reward him for what he has done" (Proverbs 19:17).

"He who oppresses the poor shows contempt for their Maker, but whoever is kind to the needy honors God" (Proverbs 14:31).

"Religion that God our Father accepts as pure and faultless is this: to look after orphans and widows in their distress and to keep oneself from being polluted by the world" (James 1:27).

David Caes and Kathleen Hayes, in their uncompromising book, *Upholding the Vision,* describe a concept which applies to our profession:

"Christian dentists and dental students need to keep in mind that their primary calling is to faith in Christ, and dentistry is a secondary calling. Most of us entered this profession as a result of a desire to serve, but sometimes the pressures of family, civic responsibilities, and other demands on us lead us to lose sight of our original motivation. We all lead very busy lives, which often lead us to neglect Bible study, and time spent alone with God. We dare not neglect these aspects of our faith, but we also dare not neglect the clear mandate in Scripture to practice our faith in our profession, by devoting some time to charitable treatment."[2]

1 John 3:17 says,

"If anyone has material possessions and sees his brother in need but has no pity on him, how can the love of God be in him? Dear children, let us not love with words or tongue, but with actions and in truth."

With *actions*. It is, in truth, a very tough standard.

The Cost

Admittedly, obedience to God's commands regarding the poor is difficult, because it is expensive to run our practices. Maintaining modern equipment is a big expense, and staff members expect to be paid a competitive salary with benefits. And the government adds to the load with requirements that often seem senseless. Despite our best efforts to keep our fees reasonable, they may seem expensive to the patient at the desk. Very often, he or she is struggling with limited resources and myriad dental problems.

As well, we dentists have a unique problem: If we become known in our communities as the one dentist who takes Medicaid, we may be overwhelmed by those patients. Yet Medicaid fees will not even cover our overhead. George Rust has written a chapter in the book *Upholding the Vision* in which he deals with this problem. Dr. Rust is a physician, a family practitioner who serves on the medical practice faculty at Morehouse School of Medicine in Atlanta. He lists three ideas whereby a physician is able to help the poor. These principles apply to dentistry as well:

God has high and specific expectations for the people who call themselves by His name.

(1) Accept new Medicaid patients. Treat the Medicaid card as if it were a gold MasterCard. "Now that's a radical idea! After all, it's harder to get a Medicaid card than a MasterCard," he says.

(2) Let your charity grow as your practice grows.

(3) Find out who does the bulk of the health care for the poor in your area, and befriend them. Offer to take their referrals willingly. They can screen out those who are not poor or those who do not really need your specialty. *Literally, be their friend*—they have a lonely job.[3]

It has become clear that the government is not going to address the needs of the poor/needs of the practitioner when it comes to dentistry. The Clinton healthcare plan, even when it was in its formative stages, barely addressed dentistry. In the state in which I practiced, the Medicaid fee schedule had not increased in ten years, and when it was implemented it was only designed to cover the dentist's costs. So the government is not going to respond to our poor patients' needs.

But the government does not have a biblical mandate to do so.

We do.

Many dentists have protocols in their own practices whereby they treat, at little or no fee, those people identified as disadvantaged and disenfranchised.

Professional Examples

The concept of sacrifice in order to aid the poor is one of our profession exhortations as well. *The Christian Medical & Dental Associations' Study Guide on Health Care for the Poor* states:

> "God has high and specific expectations for the people who call themselves by His name. Among these is that we be merciful—that is, that we possess a compassionate feeling toward those in need or distress, coupled with an active effort to meet their need or relieve their distress. Such mercy is not optional for a Christian. It is specifically commanded in Scripture and must be considered an inevitable manifestation of the saving knowledge of the Lord Jesus Christ."[4]

The Domestic Mission Commission (DMC) of CMDA was formed in 1986 to address the healthcare needs of the poor and the uninsured in the United States. At the CMDA Annual Conference in 1991, more than one hundred healthcare professionals committed to reaching out to those in need in their communities. The DMC has set a goal of facilitating as many as five clinics per year in the U.S.—fifty over the next ten years. All of these will need dental personnel.

On a broader scale, the Global Health Outreach (GHO) program sends dentists and physicians to many different countries, where poor people without access to care are treated without charge. Many of these projects are in such remote places that the only dental service provided is extractions. Other projects go to places where dental clinics are equipped with various types of operative equipment.

Most CMDA member dentists take very seriously their responsibilities as healthcare providers to the poor. Many dentists have protocols in their own practices whereby they treat, at little or no fee, those people identified as disadvantaged and disenfranchised. In most areas, there simply are not adequate public funds to pay these dentists for addressing even the most basic dental needs. In recent years, as Human Services funds in many state and federal programs have diminished, charitable services have become increasingly important.

The Position Statement of the Christian Medical & Dental Associations says:

> "Christian healthcare professionals possess a diverse array of skills, talents, and resources and are able to provide medical and surgical services, consultation, counseling, teaching, organizational leadership, and financial resources. Similarly, the Lazaruses at our doorsteps present themselves in many diverse forms. Christians are compelled to identify their own unique gifts and call to ministry. Forms of ministry may vary, but the obligation to serve with compassion is mandatory, not optional."[5]

As Christian healthcare professionals, we have a unique opportunity to fulfill Christ's commandment to love our neighbors as ourselves.

Dentistry is a noble profession. We are called upon to treat and prevent pain on a scale which most people can only dream about. Literally, we have healing potential in our hands. Dentistry can be challenging, frustrating, discouraging and extremely difficult—yet also immensely rewarding. To maintain that balance between struggle and satisfaction, we must keep sight of our original motivation—to serve humankind, be the patient wealthy or poor. To do so, in the Lord's eyes, is both biblical and the burden of proof that we are His.

Notes

1. Peter A. Boelens Jr., *Health Care for the Poor* (Richardson, Texas: Christian Medical & Dental Society, 1990).
2. David Caes and Kathleen Hayes, *Upholding the Vision* (Philadelphia: Christian Community Health Fellowship, 1993).
3. Ibid.
4. Boelens Jr., *Health Care for the Poor.*
5. Ibid.

CHAPTER SEVEN

The Place of Missions in the Life of the Dental Student and Dentist

Dental missions gives an opportunity to share in the adventure of helping change the world by following Christ's example of helping people both physically and spiritually.

Ken Chapman, D.D.S., and Richard G. Topazian, D.D.S.

Most people choose dentistry as a career because they desire to serve people and to help improve the health of humankind. These ideals of service are freshest within the dental student who is just beginning to explore the different realms of service his or her skills will open. These students ask the question, "How can I help others through dentistry?" Such a person may even consider one of the greatest ways to meet health needs by asking a more specific question, "What place should missions have in my life?"

Those who have decided to follow Christ realize that, for them, missions is not an option, but rather an essential part of their lives. After all, the final command of the Master was to go into all the world and preach the Good News. The only real questions are *how* one's particular gift of professional skills can best be applied, and *where* they can be used most effectively.

As people who have personally wrestled with these questions and experienced missions as dentists we offer the following thoughts.

The only real questions are how *one's particular gift of professional skills can best be applied, and* where *they can be used most effectively.*

Why Serve?

For the Christian, the basis for missions is the belief that peace with God is man's deepest need and the knowledge that all people need to hear God's plan of salvation, which will meet that need. The biblical foundation for this belief is found in Romans 10:13-15:

> "'Every one who calls upon the name of the Lord will be saved.' How, then can they call on the one they have not believed in? And how can they believe in the one of whom they have not heard? And how can they hear without someone preaching to them? And how can they preach unless they are sent?"

All of us who are Christians have been sent as a result of Christ's specific command and commission:

> "Go and make disciples of all nations, baptizing them in the name of the Father and of the Son and of the Holy Spirit" (Matthew 28:19).

> "You will be my witnesses in Jerusalem, and in all Judea and Samaria, and to the ends of the earth" (Acts 1:8).

It is clear from these Scriptures that making disciples is within every Christian's field of duty. But the Christian health practitioner may receive these commands with a special force, especially as he or she reads:

"Heal the sick, raise the dead, cleanse those
who have leprosy, drive out demons. Freely you
have received, freely give" (Matthew 10:8).

We read in Luke that Jesus sent the disciples "to
preach the kingdom of God and to heal the sick"
(Luke 9:2). Therefore, as Christian dentists, we are
obligated not only to make disciples but to use our
special skills of healing for the kingdom as well.

As Christian dentists, we are obligated not only to make disciples but to use our special skills of healing for the kingdom as well.

The Christian doctor's commitment to God gives
a standard by which to judge each opportunity that
presents itself; the Gospel influences the way in which
the doctor views the problems of the world. Christians
want to fulfill the commandment, "Love the Lord your
God with all your heart," and they want to express
their love for God by acts of service to others. The
Christian doctor has been given a great many talents,
and therefore, much is expected (Luke 12:48).

Have you ever dreamed that your life would
make a difference in the world at large? Dental missions gives an opportunity to share in the adventure of
helping change the world by following Christ's example of helping people both physically and spiritually.
Why not go where the need is great and your influence is unmatched?

Many missionaries and national church workers
will attest to the fact that dentistry is one of the most
needed of health services. In some places, it is the
biggest health need of all. It is all too easy in America
to minimize this need while we live in a country where
such health care is readily available.

Uganda, where Ken practices as a missionary
dentist, for example, has about one hundred dentists
for 18 million people. Most of those dentists are in the
city of Kampala, and many of them are working at limited capacity due to a lack of adequate supplies and
equipment. That works out to one dentist for every
180,000 people, and the ratio is worse in the rest of
the country. There are areas where one million people
are without a single dentist. Yet Uganda is better off
than some countries.

Imagine how it would be to live in a rural area
where the nearest dental care is ten or twenty miles

away—and you may have to walk. When you get there the only treatment offered is tooth extraction. You hope it will be done with benefit of anesthetic, but anesthetic is not always available. You hope the procedure will be done by a qualified person. Restorative care is essentially unavailable.

To make matters worse, due to scarcity of dentists, dental disease is often left untreated until it has progressed to an unbearable state for the patient, who then comes for treatment. It is a common occurrence to have patients come in with severe odontogenic infections involving the deep fascial spaces. Some of these infections are life-threatening, yet there are few if any specialists to provide treatment. Children often have severe infections. Oral tumors are sometimes left untreated until they become quite large. Acute ulcerative gingivitis is more common in many developing countries than in America. Clearly the lack of dentists in Uganda results in suffering for many people.

There are many patients for whom relatively simple dental care can make a big difference.

In Ken's clinic, however, the majority of dental disease treated is similar to what is seen in the United States. Caries and periodontal disease are the most common problems, followed by traumatic injuries. Fortunately the caries rate nationwide is not very high. Orthodontic problems are not as common as in the USA, yet there is a large demand for such services and there are few dentists who do orthodontics. In fact, there is no practicing orthodontist in Uganda.

There are many patients for whom relatively simple dental care can make a big difference. Composite restorations can transform a young girl with teeth that are unattractive due to caries or congenital malformation. A patient with a carious tooth may come expecting extraction but be happily surprised to find that the tooth can be saved.

In addition to the hundred or so dentists in Uganda, there are trained people known as Public Health Dental Assistants who have undergone a three-year course in basic dentistry. The school to train these personnel was started around 1970 to help fill the gap caused by a lack of dentists. They are taught to do extractions, class I and V restorations, prophylaxis and health education. About ten graduate annually. A dental school started in 1982 graduates about eight dentists each year.

Unfortunately, most of these dental health providers end up in the cities, many in the capital city of Kampala, while many hospitals in rural areas do not have either a dentist or a public health dental assistant. Some go in search of greener pastures in other countries, where salaries are much higher. Others end up in business, since getting equipment and supplies is difficult and expensive because almost everything has to be brought in from outside the country. All of this adds to the shortage of dentists and dental care in Uganda.

Compassionate care prepares patients for a sympathetic hearing of the Gospel.

One missionary dentist said, "I decided that one more dentist in Mississippi would not make much difference, but one more in the Ivory Coast would." Being a dentist in a country with very few dentists allows you to have an impact which would be difficult to match if you were in the United States, where there are so many more dentists.

That impact includes helping to save the lives of patients with life-threatening infections who do not have access to dental care. General dentists often end up providing care for such patients overseas due to the dearth of specialists available. You have the opportunity to provide pain-free treatment for patients who have been accustomed to having tooth extractions with no anesthetic. Now that makes an impact!

Where Does Dentistry Fit into Missions?

But how, you wonder, does dentistry advance the cause of the Gospel? It does so in the following ways:

- It is part of the general outreach ministry of healing, and it helps complete the range of health services provided through missionary medicine.

- Because of the universality of dental disease, nearly everyone is a candidate for dental services; therefore, the influence of the missionary dentist is widespread.

• Compassionate care prepares patients for a sympathetic hearing of the Gospel. Many who would not hear other missionaries will listen to those providing health care.

• It promotes a climate which is conducive to receiving the Gospel from other missionaries and national Christians.

• It is a very practical display of the love of God and the concern of Christians for serving in His name.

• It supports the Christian missionary endeavor by treating the missionary community overseas. Teachers serve missions when they teach missionary children, and missionary aviators serve in much the same way. So do missionary dentists.

We've seen the spiritual impact firsthand. Ken prays with most of his patients before treating them. This has given him the opportunity to talk to many of them about spiritual things. In a few cases, patients have prayed to invite Christ into their lives right in the dental chair. Most people in Uganda are open to talking about Christ even if they are not ready to make a commitment.

Ken remembers sharing Christ with one patient who had oral candidiasis and a generally weak appearance. She indicated a decision to receive Christ. Once he talked to a hospital patient who was so weak he couldn't speak. But he could listen as Ken shared John 3:16 with him and asked him if he wanted to accept Christ. He nodded his head. Later that night he died. More recently, Ken was sharing in the hospital, and a lady came up and said, "We also want to hear the Word of God." So he went and shared with her and her sister. It turned out that the lady herself had recently come to Christ, but her sister had not yet done so. That night her sister indicated a decision for Christ.

Ken prays with most of his patients before treating them. This has given him the opportunity to talk to many of them about spiritual things.

There can also be opportunities to be a witness to your local dental colleagues and other professionals through involvement in dental societies, civic organizations and so on. Serving as vice-president, secretary, and president of the Uganda Dental Association has given Ken contact with many Ugandan colleagues. He has been active in a local church which has helped him grow spiritually and given him opportunities for outreach.

Your ministry as a dentist can also help give credibility to the mission or organization for which you are working, by providing physical services to the people. Many governments are interested primarily in the physical help that you or your mission can offer. In some countries, the only way missionaries can get in is by being able to provide such a service to the people. Dentistry may open a door which a traditional missionary can no longer get through.

Dentistry may open a door which a traditional missionary can no longer get through.

Where and How Can I Serve?

God has called all Christians to be His witnesses; the Christian dentist has unique skills and opportunities to do so. Therefore, the remaining question is, "Where and how does God want to use me?" The options for service are many. Most dentists do not find it possible to serve as full-time missionaries at the onset of their careers, although this possibility should be prayerfully considered.

In the United States, most dentists can find, within an office or clinic, many occasions to serve others and to share their faith. Opportunities exist beyond the office also, through serving in local areas where the dental needs rival the needs overseas. Many dentists participate in mission projects in their own towns and cities. Some provide free care to poor patients and to Christian missionaries. Some offer service in prisons or mission clinics.

In addition to service at home, personal involvement in missions abroad, where the need is overwhelming and therefore the impact is greatest, is one of the most fulfilling and spiritually enriching experiences one can have. Tithing one's time through short-term, one- to two-week projects annually can fit well with the obligations of an active practice. There are many such opportunities available through CMDA and other groups.

Several agencies such as those noted below provide well-organized projects where dental skills may be put to immediate and effective use. Spouses and teenage children may often share in this work, strengthening bonds with each other as well as serving others together. Short-term experiences will often lead to involvement for longer periods of time. A number of dentists, after participating in two-week projects annually for some years, have left practice for full-time service overseas as they have come to see how much more effective they can be when on the field for longer periods.

A trend in recent years is to serve after retirement or early retirement (hence the title "second-career missionary"). Mature missionary dentists and their spouses can have a most beneficial effect in the place of service, not only with their professional skills, but as mentors and counselors to younger missionaries and their children.

Career dental missionaries often have an impact on the dental health of a locale or a large region as they provide leadership for dental health measures such as fluoride treatment, oral hygiene and similar concerns.

The impact that missionary dentists can have on local missionaries is very special. The treatment they provide to other missionaries allows them to remain on the field without expensive trips home or to other countries to get needed dental work. Some missionary dentists provide orthodontic services for the children of missionaries who would otherwise have some difficult decisions to make as to how and if their children can be treated.

One area of impact often not considered is in providing dental care for the more affluent people in the country—diplomats, business people, government officials and the like. Ken has seen patients from well over thirty countries and from many walks of life in his practice in Uganda, including ambassadors and high government officials. In some cases he has had the

One area of impact often not considered is in providing dental care for the more affluent people in the country—diplomats, businesspeople and government officials.

chance to share spiritual things with such people. They come to him—he doesn't have to go out and look for them! In many countries, people like these are not well reached with the Gospel, yet they wield great influence in the society. They are often open to spiritual things, yet there are few who seek to minister to them. As a professional you may have an access to them that others do not have.

As well, in some countries there is a need for qualified people to teach in local dental schools, or to start training programs where none exist. (For information about service opportunities, see the list at the end of the chapter.)

Where Do I Fit into Missions?

Take active, aggressive steps to investigate needs and opportunities for service.

You may be thinking: *I understand my responsibility before God to witness and to heal. I'm aware of the need that exists. But how do I know if missions is my specific calling?* To answer this we must first do away with the misconceptions many have about serving in missions. In his book *Myths About Missions,* Horace Fenton, of the Latin American Mission, describes some of these.[1]

Myth #1: Missions are for only a small band of spiritually elite. In truth, all Christians are called to witness; that is, to serve as missionaries, some in a home setting and others in distant parts of the world.

Myth #2: A ministry location is always final; the lifetime call is fixed and rigid. In truth, circumstances change. Changes may occur in children's educational needs, or in the care of parents. There may be special health needs or opportunities to use one's talents in a new setting. These and other factors may cause a change in location. Pastors move from one church to another, and that is not considered unusual. Similarly, missionaries may move home from the field, and they may move back to the field again.

As Fenton says, discipleship is for life, but one's location of service isn't.

Myth #3: The task of evangelizing the world is almost finished. The truth is, great strides have been made in reaching the world with the Gospel, but much remains to be done.

Myth #4. The task is unfinishable. In truth, Christ said it *would* be done, and commanded us to make it happen:

> "This gospel of the kingdom will be preached in the whole world as a testimony to all nations, and then the end will come" (Matthew 24:14).

Fenton helps us see that missions is a vital call for every generation; therefore, every disciple—dentists and dental students alike—should weigh carefully the opportunities for obeying it.

How, then, can one discern his or her own call? Some people hold the view that God leads Christians to a specific place of service. They believe that without such specificity, one has not been genuinely "called." Yet, as author Eugene Nida has said, many people find the call to missions in simply recognizing the need and applying one's abilities to meeting that need. For some it is as simple as asking, "Is there a need? Can I help fill that need?"

Make prayerful commitment to God, asking Him to confirm opportunities, and to block avenues which do not conform to His will for your life.

Other considerations in clarifying one's "calling" include the following:

First, take active, aggressive steps to investigate needs and opportunities for service. Correspond with missionary dentists. Learn how God called them to service. Learn what they do, and how it furthers God's kingdom. (CMDA can help connect you with missionary dentists—see the end of this chapter for contact information.)

Participate in missions at home or overseas during your student days. Consider spending a week or two on an overseas project or take an elective month of dental school working with a missionary dentist. One student spent a month in Africa with an American missionary dentist; this experience helped confirm God's call on the student's life for full-time service overseas. His host missionary dentist was himself called to missions through a similar experience while a dental student.

During Ken's student days, he came into contact with a group called Missionary Dentists through

InterCristo, an organization that matches people with Christian groups with which they might be able to serve. Missionary Dentists sponsored Ken on a six-week trip to Korea during the summer break between his third and fourth years in dental school. His experiences there strongly influenced him when it came time to choose between local practice or overseas work. The openness of the people to the Gospel combined with the great need for dental services in Korea at that time, as well as another short-term trip to Liberia, West Africa, inspired his eventual decision to choose career dental missions.

The Christian dentist and dental student should not necessarily expect a supernatural sign declaring his or her destiny regarding missions.

The point is, find out as much as you can, through research and personal experience, about missions. Read mission publications and attend mission conferences. One's own church publications and Christian magazines like *Today's Christian Doctor* often feature mission-related articles. Read the biographies of missionaries and books by contemporary medical missionaries, like Drs. Paul Brand and Tom Hale, and subscribe to mission publications like *Mission Frontiers* and *The Evangelical Missions Quarterly*. Attend missionary conferences such as those held by churches and denominations, and the Urbana Missions Conference conducted triennially by InterVarsity Christian Fellowship.

Second, make prayerful commitment to God, asking Him to confirm opportunities, and to block avenues which do not conform to His will for your life. This includes making, as a highest priority, a daily personal devotional time. A vital spiritual life is essential to knowing how and where God wants you to serve. It also involves worshiping regularly at a church and fellowshipping with student Christian groups. (The local chapters of Christian Medical & Dental Associations, InterVarsity Christian Fellowship and Campus Crusade for Christ are excellent.)

Third, act in submission to others; heed their advice. This is especially important for the dental student who does decide on missions. Working under the authority of a missions organization involves some loss of personal autonomy. Professionals must be willing to accept this loss "for the sake of Christ," as Paul wrote in Philippians 3:7. Choose counselors and col-

Serving Christ in missions by using the specific talent God has given you through dentistry is a most exciting and fulfilling way to live.

leagues wisely. Your choice of friends, and especially of a spouse, is vitally important in encouraging one to mission service. Make friends of people who are open to God's leading, especially with regard to missionary service.

Fourth, handle money wisely. (See chapter nine.) Avoid nonessential debt and other encumbrances which may deflect you from your goal of serving in missions. Taking on the trappings of the consumer-oriented American lifestyle will diminish your appetite for service, and can load you with debt. Perhaps more than anything, debt can prevent you from serving in some needy location.

Finally, the Christian dentist and dental student should not necessarily expect a supernatural sign declaring his or her destiny regarding missions. We should remember that men and women with no religious motivation will leave home, family, and friends, risking disease and disaster in many places around the globe for financial gain or adventure. Those of us who believe people are lost without the Gospel should be at least as motivated. We should not expect a dramatic or miraculous "call" before leaving the security of home.

It is much more simple: If the Christian dentist or dental student finds a match between the world's needs and his or her skills, is suited for the special demands of missions work, has consulted wise counsel in coming to this decision, and senses definitely the Lord's confirmation of this choice, he or she should identify sending agencies and begin to prepare for an appointment. It's no good to say, "I'll go where You want me to go, dear Lord," and then proceed with other plans. Writing of such persons, Robertson McQuilken states in *The Great Omission*, "They are willing to go, but planning to stay." Actively plan to go to the field, and proceed unless the Lord raises barriers to this course of action.

Getting some experience after dental school as an associate in practice or in a residency program before leaving for career overseas work is most valuable. Take advantage of opportunities for spiritual training as well. Some mission organizations provide excellent programs to help prepare candidates.

Training in evangelism and discipleship, Bible study, and prayer also prove invaluable.

Serving Christ in missions by using the specific talent God has given you through dentistry is a most exciting and fulfilling way to live. Whether this service is at home or abroad, it will provide an enduring and abundant spiritual, professional and personal life. The plan under which we operate—the "Great Commission"—has been called the greatest plan ever given to men, by the greatest person who ever lived, concerning the greatest power ever revealed, and with the greatest promise ever recorded.

As Christians, we are a sent people, a people with a mission. As Christian dentists, we are a sent people with healing in our hands, for both the body and the spirit. Combining a spiritual ministry and a physical one such as dentistry follows the example of our Lord Jesus Christ, who went about healing and preaching the Gospel. It is, we can say from experience, a glorious combination!

Notes

1. Horace L. Fenton, *Myths About Missions* (Downers Grove, IL: InterVarsity Press, 1973).

Suggested Reading

Paul Borthwick. *A Mind for Missions.* Colorado Springs: NavPress, 1988.

Thomas Hale. *On Being a Missionary.* Pasadena, CA: William Carey Library, 1995.

Robertson McQuilkin. *The Great Omission.* Grand Rapids: Baker Book House,1984.

Eugene A. Nida. *Message and Mission. The Communication of the Christian Faith* . Pasadena, CA: William Carey Library, 1990.

Marion and Robert Schindler. *Mission Possible.* Wheaton: Victor Books, 1984.

David S. Topazian. *God's Prescription for Your Finances.* Richardson, Texas: Christian Medical & Dental Society, 1992.

Evangelical Missions Quarterly, P.O. Box 794,
Wheaton, IL 60189.
Missions Frontiers, U.S. Center for World Mission,
1605 Elizabeth, Pasadena, CA 91104.

Opportunities

For more information about opportunities for missionary dentistry, short- or long-term, contact:

InterCristo
19303 Fremont Ave., North
Seattle, WA 98133
1-800-251-7740
Web site: http://www.lcyon.com/ico/links.html.

Christian Dental Society
P.O. Box 177
Sumner, IA 50674
1-800-237-7368

Global Health Outreach
Christian Medical and Dental Associations
P.O. Box 7500
Bristol, TN 37621-7500
Phone: (423) 844-1000; Fax: (423) 844-1005
Web site: http://www.cmdahome.org

Medical Ministry International
P.O. Box 940207
Plano, TX 75094-0207
(972) 437-1995
Web site: http://www.mmint.org

CHAPTER EIGHT

Dental Marriages: Their Stresses and Strengths

Wise dentists blend their own strengths with the strengths of their spouses in managing life's stresses.

Lewis Penhall Bird, S.T.M., Ph.D.

People who marry usually hope that their mutual joy will last forever and presume that the public ceremony merely sanctions what is already assumed. Dentists who marry usually hope, in addition, that the constraints of their healthcare careers will be less demanding than those of their physician colleagues, for example, and presume that their private lives will be similar to other upper-middle-class neighbors. Christians who marry usually hope, further, that their relationships have been directed and blessed by a covenant-keeping God of love and grace and presume thereby that their vows are "'til death do us part."

In building the marital relationship, each couple brings to this task their own unique personalities, their own unique styles, their particular vulnerabilities.

And in the construction of this covenantal bond, each couple will have to cultivate the universal skills of communication, problem solving, financial management, mutual sensitivity and conflict resolution. In these tasks, dental marriages differ from no others.

Dental personalities have been studied, from dental-school days into the midlife years, and we can learn from this research.

But if certain personality types are attracted to dentistry, are there distinctive strengths and weaknesses that these individuals bring to marriage that are particularly noteworthy? For the dental student already married or considering marriage, are there relationship issues unique to his or her profession? We will address these questions in this chapter. First, let us look at the personalities most prone to study dentistry and how they play out in marriage.

Dental Personalities

Vibrant, vivacious personalities appear in every profession; withdrawn, neurotic people make their appearances as well. Bell-shaped curves preserve the middle range for the typical types. Fortunately, dental personalities have been studied, from dental-school days into the midlife years, and we can learn from this research. A 1963 study described aspects of the typical dental student. Some were attributes devoutly to be wished for by patients ("persistent, conscientious, methodical, neat and orderly, interested in applied rather than theoretical knowledge") but others were problematic for marital relationships ("conventional, unconsciously aggressive, somewhat rigid and inflexible, nonintrospective").[1] Obviously at issue here is: What personal traits belong in the office and which ones enhance a marriage? How does one maximize certain attributes in the right setting, and modify other traits in other situations?

To help us answer these questions, we must look to more recent data. The most popular survey instrument in the past few decades appears to be the Myers-Briggs Type Indicator (MBTI). The MBTI measures characteristics under two headings: 1) Mental Attitudes, including extroversion (E) or introversion (I) and judgment (J) or perception (P), and 2) Mental Functions, including sensing (S) or intuition (N) and thinking (T) or feeling (F).[2] Using the MBTI instrument in the early 1980s to evaluate dental students at the University of Mississippi, Silberman et al. found five personality types (ESFJ, ESTJ, ISFJ, ISTJ, and ENFJ) constituting 53 percent of this population. Among these top five personality types, dental students consistently rated higher in the sensing and judging characteristics. Noteworthy also, the judging trait dominated in all five types over the perceptive trait. Compared to the general population, a disproportionately low number of intuitive types appeared as well.[3]

These findings have implications for marital interactions. Reflection on the top two personality classifications (which were the only ones Silberman et al. reflected on) could be particularly useful in understanding interpersonal interactions.

1. The ISFJ Personality Type

These persons "are concerned chiefly with people. They see themselves as exuding qualities of warmth, sympathy, tactfulness, and friendliness. . . . They consider differing views wrong or unimportant. They see themselves as persevering, conscientious, and orderly, and they tend to want others to be the same."[4]

Such dentists are marriage partners who will usually bring emotional warmth and empathic companionship to a relationship, but who may appear to be intolerant of opinions or decisions which differ from their own. They may be overly perfectionistic about home decor and family behaviors. As with other professionals who live very demanding, highly stressful lives in the office, the dentist needs to analyze very carefully his or her personality traits, bring to patient care those skills most admirable there and modify in marital life those traits which could be very destructive in that context.

2. The ESTJ Personality Type

These individuals "tend to use thinking to run their lives and are concerned with impersonal truth, thought-out plans, and orderly efficiency. These persons view themselves as being analytical, impersonal,

Among these top five personality types, dental students consistently rated higher in the sensing and judging characteristics.

and objectively critical. They like to run things, put themselves into their job, and insist on order, rules, and logic . . . however, they seem to need intuitive types around them to sell them on the value of new ideas."[5]

As marriage partners, these dentists may overintellectualize problems, relying on the cerebral in relationships but exhibiting little empathy or warmth in marital interactions. Their need to control can be ruinous unless traits appropriate to the office are strongly modified in a marriage so that complementary insights can be respected and viewed as necessary and appropriate. Partnership in marriage is well-managed where each spouse contributes in areas of strength, is truly heard, and decisions are mutually agreed-upon.

The Silberman study concluded that these personalities exhibited "a significantly high need for order, resulting in a lack of spontaneity and flexibility."[6] Often the traits lacking in the dentist can be found in the spouse and are, in fact, part of the attraction that drew the couple together in the first place. If "opposites attract" (and there is some justification for such a hypothesis), then spousal traits can aid in modifying and balancing dental characteristics so that harmonious living is possible. Obviously, where traits clash rather than mesh, conflict is inevitable.

The bad news, then, is, that the personality characteristics of those drawn to the field of dentistry can be useful in the office but problematic at home. But the good news is that dentists are quite intelligent people with a marked capacity for empathy, and cultivating the skill to be trait-appropriate in the clinical setting or in the home is well within their reach. Where the love of Christ constrains any one of us, sensitivity, compassion and sympathy for the struggles and accomplishments of others can characterize any Christian dentist. And, since all of us live with our own particular vulnerabilities, wounds and dark sides, we're fortunate that the grace of God can cultivate our finer traits where we are willing to grow and to transform our worst characteristics where we are too weak to change.

Dentists who are people-oriented have the

capacity to find their professional focus in the Golden Rule. (Dentists who are power- and wealth-oriented are usually interested in the rule of gold.) Beyond personality lies the grander vision of virtue and character; therein lies excellence in patient care and ultimate service to the Lord God, with Whom we all have our appointed destiny. Therein lies marital happiness as well; and this brings us to dental marriages.

Dental Marriages

What do we know of dental marriages? To be honest, not much information is available. At the outset of the 1990s, the American Dental Association could report that:

> "Among dentists generally, slightly more than 2 percent of male dentists are married to other dentists, while nearly 30 percent of female dentists find themselves with a dental partner in marriage. But among dentists younger than 30, nearly 4 percent of males and 31 percent of females are married to dentists."[7]

Sixty-six percent of the wives [who responded to the survey] described their marriage as "above average . . ."

Beyond these data on dual-career dental marriages, little seems to be known other than anecdotal impressions. Still, given the problems all professional marriages encounter these days, even if data is scarce, it is relevant to use what is available.

One dentist's wife sent a questionnaire on "Life as the Wife of a Dentist" to 350 dentists' wives in Northern Virginia. With a 40-percent response, she drew these conclusions concerning dentists and marriage:

First, dentists do not have a high rate of divorce. Of the respondents, 76 percent were the first wife. National statistics indicate that nearly 50 percent of American marriages end in divorce, so the marriages of dentists surveyed are more durable than the average marriage. Sixty-six percent of the wives described their marriage as "above average," 25 percent as "average" and only 9 percent as "poor." Asked whether they were disappointed in their life as the wife of a dentist, 16 percent answered "yes." Their causes

of disappointment were twofold: they had not anticipated the stress of dentistry, and they had expected
greater financial returns.[8]

**Second, there are approximately six areas of
stress in a dental marriage.** These are: time and
energy depletion; personal anxieties with business
stress; lack of adequate communication with the marital partner; power strains between appropriate office
and home roles; financial problems; child-rearing
problems—particularly in the teenage years.

In explanation, a recent brief article in *The Wall
Street Journal* described the typical dentist as outgoing, well-organized and concerned about details. To
spouses, who see these qualities not in a quick inter-
view but in years of living together, "concerned about
details" is "perfectionist." "Well-organized" carried to
its extreme is "compulsive" and "outgoing" can easily
become over-involvement in social and civic activities,
or even "social climbing."

Nearly half of the wives who responded to the
survey mentioned above agreed that there is such a
thing as a "dental personality." [Still], "for every wife
who confided, 'I wouldn't marry a dentist again,' there
were five who said, 'Our life together gets better all
the time.'"[9]

> *Nearly half of the
> wives surveyed
> agreed that there is
> such a thing as a
> "dental personality."*

Personal Observations

Having enjoyed the dividends of over thirty-five
years living in a marriage truly crafted in heaven, and
having worked shoulder to shoulder for over thirty-two
years with dental and medical colleagues in the
Christian Medical & Dental Associations, I have few
observations to add here.

Clearly, given the time, income, and inclination of medical and dental personnel, there is no limit
to the mischief and dysfunction that can be created by
disaffected spouses; after all, these are "above-average" (high-achieving) individuals.

Given the increasingly obvious dividends of
building a mutually satisfying relationship, of con-

fronting and solving life's problems, of supporting and encouraging one another in reaching our God-endowed potential and of discovering the pleasure derived from building a home together, marital happiness can be one of life's choicest rewards.

Given a commitment to pursuing God's will in marriage, the riches of faith, hope, and love are to be treasured far beyond any quest for power, control and wealth. Eternal values really are transcendent and the values of this world really are counterfeit.

In brief, we have a goal—a happy and satisfying Christian marriage—that will be attacked, but that is also worth fighting for.

Wisdom about marriage shines through the conclusions of the classic analysis of *The Mirages of Marriage*. Its authors describe the characteristics of smooth-running marriage:

The fact that marriages are more enduring when both partners have focused faith is well-supported in the literature.

"First, the spouses in a workable marriage respect each other. The greater the number of areas of respect, the more satisfactory is the marriage.

Second, the spouses are tolerant of each other. They see themselves as fallible, vulnerable human beings and can therefore accept each other's shortcomings.

Third, the key ingredient in a successful marriage is the effort of the spouses to make the most of its assets and minimize its liabilities."[10]

From experience and data, I can assure you that the grace of God is a very powerful support for Christian couples in conforming to these standards.

Christian Marriages

The fact that marriages are more enduring when both partners have focused faith is well-supported in the literature.[11] While it is true that some spouses stay together in response to their church's prohibitions regarding divorce, more evidence exists to suggest that marital satisfaction measurements for this group routinely transcend the average in various studies. The Glenn and Weaver study disclosed that church attendance alone as a modest measurement predicted marital satisfaction far better than any of the other eight variables.[12] In the analysis of Sporawski and Houghston, men and women in enduring marriages consistently rank religious commitment as one of the most important ingredients in a happy marriage.[13] In his extensive survey of studies that associate religious involvement with marital status, marital well-being, and mortality, David Larson concludes:

> "The evidence . . . suggests that one's religious commitment is positively associated with the maintaining of a marriage. In addition, higher degrees of religious commitment are associated with more satisfied marriages and lower death rate—even after adjusting for the appropriate ris factors."[14]

Summing up over two decades of an enduring, happy marriage as well as two decades of research on marriage, Larson and his wife, Susan, offer ten summary qualities of enduring marriages:

1. Commitment—to each other and to the marriage.
2. Wise decision making.
3. Trust.
4. Shared values.
5. An assumption of permanence.
6. Good communication.
7. Acceptance and adaptability.
8. Shared emotional interdependence and appreciation of each other.
9. Intimacy.
10. A sense of humor.[15]

Christian marriages are central to the diversity of American religiously-oriented marriages evaluated by these investigators. At the heart of any Christian marriage is a sense of covenantal bonding that originates in the God of Christian life, Himself, and extends to the couple both in their marriage and in

At the heart of any Christian marriage is a sense of covenantal bonding that originates in the God of Christian life, Himself, and extends to the couple both in their marriage and in their family life.

their family life. The dual themes—marriage is honorable and marriage is for life—ring in the ears of Christians who are married. For those who actively cultivate the fruit of the Spirit in their lives together, nine virtues undergird the marriage in a way that is both enhancing and remedial: love, joy, peace, patience, kindness, goodness, fidelity, gentleness and self-control. Happy is the couple where each is governed thereby.

As an addendum to this section, let me express my opinion that for the contemporary Christian couple that there two paradigms for Christian marriages: namely, the male leadership model[16] and the equalitarian model.[17] Many modern Christian couples find themselves afflicted with theological schizophrenia as they move back and forth between the university and the church, between equal opportunities in the workplace and often-presumed male leadership at home and in the church. Serious reflection may be necessary in those contemporary marriages where issues of power, roles and decision making are unresolved or ill-resolved, where each partner sincerely wishes to honor Christ and honor his or her partner. Each couple needs to develop their own theology of Christian marriage. Some couples know and accept the male leadership model, while others may wish to adopt a more equalitarian approach. What remains is for each couple to do their homework and to discover for themselves God's plan for them. In either model Christ may be present and in either home strangers may be refreshed.

Careers have their own satisfactions, but it is in the daily give and take of a solid marriage, where one is cherished and challenged to grow, that personal maturity has its finest moments.

Conclusion

As we have seen, in some ways dental marriages and dental home lives are unique; in most ways they are similar to professional colleagues from a rainbow of careers. Wise dentists read the studies and read the faces of those dearest to them and then pray that Almighty God will energize both their resources and their resolve to be worthy of the titles "Sweetheart" and "Beloved." Paul Tournier described the traits needed for any successful marriage (whether including that of a dentist and spouse or not):

Wise dentists blend their own strengths with the strengths of their spouses in managing life's stresses.

"He who loves understands, and he who understands loves. One who feels understood feels loved, and one who feels loved feels sure of being understood. Deep sharing is overwhelming, and very rare. No one can develop freely in this world and find a full life without feeling understood by at least one person. Alone, a man marks time and becomes very set in his ways. In the demanding confrontation which marriage constitutes, he must ever go beyond himself, develop, grow up into maturity."[8]

Careers have their own satisfactions, but it is in the daily give and take of a solid marriage, where one is cherished and challenged to grow, that personal maturity has its finest moments. Dentists certainly have many personal strengths which can enhance a marriage. Wise dentists blend their own strengths with the strengths of their spouses in managing life's stresses. The wisest seek the grace of God to remain faithful to those original vows. When Scripture says, "Marriage is honorable; let us all keep it so" (Hebrews 13:4 NEB), the larger context urges us to seek the grace of God whenever this honor is in jeopardy.

Notes

1. J. H. Manhold, L. Shatin, and B. S. Manhold, "Comparison of Interests, Needs, and Selected Personality Factors of Dental and Medical Students," *Journal of the American Dental Association* 67 (1963): 601-5.
2. I. B. Myers, *The Myers-Briggs Type Indicator* (Palo Alto: Consulting Psychologists Press, 1962).
3. S. L. Silberman, M. J. Cain, and J. M. Mahan, "Dental Students' Personality: A Jungian Perspective," *Journal of Dental Education* 46 (1982): 646-51.
4. Ibid.
5. Ibid.
6. Ibid.
7. Cited in David O. Born, "Dentists Married to Dentists," *Journal of the American Dental*

Association 122 (1991): 67-9.

8. E. Hines, and I. H. Humphrey, "The Myths of Dental Marriages," *TIC* 45 (1986): 9-12.

9. Ibid.

10. William J. Lederer and Don D. Jackson, *The Mirages of Marriage* (New York: W. W. Norton & Co., Inc., 1968), 198.

11. Cited in George Rekers, ed., *Family Building* (Ventura, CA.: Regal Books, l985), 121-147.

12. N. D. Glenn and C. N. Weaver, "A Multivariate, Multi-Survey Study of Marital Happiness," *Journal of Marriage & Family* 40 (1978): 269-82.

13. M. J. Sporawski and M. J. Houghston, "Prescriptions for Happy Marriage Adjustments and Satisfaction of Couples Married 50 or More Years," *Family Coordinator* 27 (1978): 321-27.

14. Rekers, *Family Building*, 121-147.

15. Cited in John Gartner, ed., *Behavior and Medicine* (New York: Mosby Yearbook, 1990), pp. 138ff.

16. Cf. Lawrence J. Crabbe, Jr., *The Marriage Builder* (Grand Rapids: Zondervan, 1982) and James H. Olthius, *I Pledge You My Troth* (New York: Harper and Row, 1975).

17. Cf. Alvera Mickelsen, ed., *Women, Authority & the Bible* (Downers Grove, IL: InterVarsity Press, 1986) and Mary Stewart Van Leeuwen, *Gender and Grace* (Downers Grove, IL: InterVarsity Press, 1990).

18. Paul Tournier, *To Understand Each Other*, trans. John S. Gilmour (Richmond: John Knox Press, 1967), 28ff.

CHAPTER NINE

Financial Issues for the Christian Dentist:
Money Management, Debt, Tithing

Probably all of us are very rich by the world's standards. It is our obligation to generously share what we have and be certain that we are doing good works, not for our salvation, but as a means of truly enjoying both this life and the next.

David S. Topazian, D.D.S., M.B.A.

Several years ago at my specialty society convention, I hailed a contemporary of mine, who quickly backed me into a corner and started peppering me with questions. "I heard that you were retiring to do missionary work. How can you retire at your age? Does mission work pay that well?"

"No, it doesn't pay well at all," I responded. "I am going as an unpaid volunteer, working for the Lord." My colleague then pushed me further into the corner and dissected my financial life and history, wanting to know every detail about my pension fund, the value of my home, the buyout arranged with my partners and so on.

"Why is this so important to you?" I asked, somewhat bewildered by the doctor's aggressiveness in relation to my private affairs.

Unfortunately, for many people, money and its acquisition become an end in themselves.

"I am older than you are and I want to retire, too," my colleague said. "The fact is, I can't retire. I don't have a cent."

Thinking that my colleague was needling me, I asked, "What about your retirement plan?"

"I never funded my plan."

"What about your savings and investments?"

"My 'ex' took half of all I owned. I wasted most of the rest at the country club. The truth is, I get up and go to work every morning because I have to, not because I want to. And I hate every minute of it." I winced, thinking about being operated on by an oral surgeon with such an attitude toward work.

I had always admired this colleague's sophistication, poise, good looks and athleticism. Because I had a rough idea of the money that had passed through this doctor's hands during at least a thirty-year career, I found it hard to believe that nothing was left.

I have since discovered that this doctor's story is not so rare. In fact, it is devastatingly common and a real tragedy. When this kind of story is told by a Christian, it is doubly tragic because the Scriptures have so much to say about money and its management. Moreover, as believers in, and followers of, Jesus Christ, we are obligated to search the Scriptures and adjust our attitudes and actions so that they are in accord with what the Bible teaches. Following biblical principles certainly should lead to solvency and financial independence after a lifetime of earning.

Attitudes about Money

First, we need to understand what money is. Money is nothing more than a medium of exchange. It is a wonderful convenience, certainly, when compared with bartering goods for goods and commodities for commodities. You put the cash in your pocket instead of taking home bales of cotton or a barrel of flour.

Money is a means to an end. It allows us to purchase the necessities of life. Unfortunately, for many people, money and its acquisition become an end in themselves, and when this happens such people have already strayed from the teachings of Scripture.

Paul the Apostle, writing to Timothy, described three classes of people in relation to their attitudes about material things.

First, there are those with few possessions, who are satisfied with what they have:

> "For we brought nothing into the world, and we can take nothing out of it. But if we have food and clothing, we will be content with that" (1 Timothy 6:6).

This group, and Paul places himself within it, consists of *those who are not rich.* To them he says, "Don't follow the false teaching that godliness is a means to financial gain." The truth is that godliness with contentment is of more worth than a lot of money that has no eternal value.

The second group that Paul identifies consists of *those who want to get rich* (verse 9). They are prone to let their appetites for the foolish and harmful things that money can buy pull them into a trap that brings ruin and destruction their way. They seem to develop a love for money that becomes a root of evil, leading them to do real harm to themselves and to wander away from their faith—the only asset that will not pass away.

Those who are rich in this present world comprise Paul's third group (vv. 17-19). He warns them not to be arrogant, nor to put their hope in wealth—wealth can quickly disappear—but to put their hope in God, Who is eternal and quite capable of supplying all our needs. Rich Christians should be generous and willing to share their money. Rich Christians should be busy doing good deeds, not just buying things to gratify themselves. Rich Christians ought to be laying up treasure as a firm foundation for eternity, and in doing so their values will be solidly based—"that they might take hold of the life that is truly life" (1 Timothy 6:19).

Where do you and I fit in Paul's classifica-

"People who want to get rich fall into temptation and . . . destruction. Command those who are rich in this present world not to be arrogant nor to put their hope in wealth, which is so uncertain, but to put their hope in God, who richly provides us with everything for our enjoyment. Command them to do good, to be rich in good deeds, and to be generous and willing to share"
(1 Timothy 6:9, 17-18).

tions? I venture to say that most of us fit in all three categories. Very few of us consider ourselves rich. Deep down, we know that we can't take our possessions with us when we die, causing us to be somewhat content with food and shelter. But at the same time, we wouldn't mind being a little richer, since we could always use a little more to pay tuition for our children's education or to buy something we really don't need but which "we deserve for working so hard." (We need to be on guard that going for that "little bit more" doesn't pull us away from our devotion to Jesus.) And probably all of us are very rich by the world's standards. We have options. Most of the world does not. That makes us rich, and it is our obligation to share generously what we have and be certain that we are doing good works, not for our salvation, but as a means of truly enjoying both this life and the next.

God owns all material things. We may possess them for a little while, but we do not own them.

Managers of God's Resources

The parable of the talents, told by Jesus in Matthew 25:14-30, provides us with some excellent principles about the importance of properly managing the material things God has entrusted to us. A master goes away on a trip. He gives some assets of different values to three managers. The first two invest and double the assets; the third, thinking only about what a difficult boss he has, plays it safe and buries the money. When the master returns, he commends the two who have invested wisely and gives them greater responsibilities. He condemns the one who buried the asset, claiming that the least the manager could have done is to have put the money in the bank, where it could have earned some interest. His condemnation is severe, and he strips the manager not only of his asset, but of future responsibilities.

In analyzing this parable we see that it emphasizes something: Verses 14, 18, and 25 make it quite clear that the master had given them *his* property to manage. This is probably the most important point of this parable, because it puts all material things in perspective. God owns all material things.

We may possess them for a little while, but we do not own them. We tacitly recognize this fact when we say, "You can't take it with you." Even though some of those things we possess will pass on to our heirs after our death, much of their value will be eaten up in taxes, and in a generation or two the home we "owned" and other things we think of as being substantive, if not permanent, probably will have passed into the ownership of total strangers.

The second principle apparent in this parable is that the amount we are given to manage is less important in God's sight than what we do with it. One manager had five talents, the second had two, and the third, one. But the managers who doubled the value of the talents both got the same commendation, namely, a "well done" plus increased responsibilities.

The third principle involves styles of management. Good stewardship requires action. Those who were active and aggressive in management were commended. The servant who "played it safe" used the excuse that he was working for a stern taskmaster and that he feared losing the principal. But he was called " wicked" and "lazy" and the little that he had was taken from him. Rather than sharing his master's happiness, he experienced only isolation and unhappiness. Passive management had made him a pauper.

Fourth, the parable makes it clear for whose benefit managers exert themselves. All of the managers acted for the benefit of the master, but in acquitting themselves well of the responsibilities placed upon them, they, as well as their master, reaped benefits. Those who were good managers shared the happiness of the master, himself.

As Christians settling accounts in eternity, we will experience no greater joy than hearing "well done" and sharing the pure happiness of our Creator, God. Nothing money can buy could afford the same pleasure.

As Christians settling accounts in eternity, we will experience no greater joy than hearing "well done" and sharing the pure happiness of our Creator, God. Nothing money can buy could afford the same pleasure.

Five Elements of Successful Financial Management

God's ownership of all material possessions is more likely to call us to a realistic distinction between needs and wants.

What ingredients create financial success? How can we who earn above-average incomes look to a future with some security while dealing day by day with increasing costs, expensive educational expenses for our children, governmental interference into our practices, the economic threat of managed care in dentistry, higher taxes and any number of other financial ogres?

Five basic principles will guarantee financial success, if adhered to diligently. Several have already been demonstrated from the Scriptures, therefore they demand our attention. The others are no more sophisticated than common sense, but most of us need to work hard at the discipline sometimes necessary to bring common-sense behavior and theory into harmony.

1. Realize that God owns everything.

In an age when autonomy is highly valued, and in times when the secular philosophy emphasizes self-fulfillment, self-development and self-gratification, it is very difficult to cede ownership of all we possess to another.

"We earned it, and we deserve it."
"If I had not made wise decisions, we wouldn't own things of such high quality."
"It's mine, and I have the right to do with it as I please."

Both Christians and nonbelievers frequently make comments like these. The problem is, when we insist on ownership, there is no accountability. We can do with it as we please. But that is not what Scripture teaches. The Christian who submits to Scripture wants to discover and embrace the plethora of managerial prescriptions in Scripture. These instructions will help us manage what is entrusted to us with the kind of wisdom only God can impart.

God's ownership of all material possessions is more likely to call us to a realistic distinction between needs and wants. We need food, clothing and shelter, all of which can be of good quality. But when we step over the line that separates needs from wants, we have subtly yearned for things that we feel we want, ought to have, or have the right to own. As one young surgeon said when trying to explain the rationale for buying a very expensive gadget, "I just like nice things."

2. See money as a tool, not a goal.

The financially bloated industrialist listened wanly as the questions came rapid-fire: "When will you have enough? You work a full day in your late eighties and are a multimultimillionaire. When will you have enough?"

In all seriousness he replied, "When I get just a little bit more."

This answer might be right for a person who is driven by money and who is in such a lofty position that he or she feels no sense of accountability. But it is not all right for the Christian. Christ should be first in our lives and a drive for more material possessions will drive Him out of the place He deserves. Pursuing wealth will trap us and destroy not only our dependence on God but our desire to serve Him.

I asked a middle-aged healthcare professional to assist in a ministry opportunity that would require one evening of activity. She told me that she had to be on call every weekend because she had such great financial needs and a daughter in college. She could not give up one night's potential income. Was she pursuing money as a goal? At the least, she had placed the possibility of earning a few dollars above an opportunity for Christian witness and service. At the worst, her attitude would ultimately close out ministry

"When you make a vow to God, do not delay in fulfilling it. He has no pleasure in fools; fulfill your vow. It is better not to vow than to make a vow and not fulfill it"
(Ecclesiastes 5:4-5).

opportunities since people, once they find a person unwilling to put Christian service in a priority position, will not usually ask again. The biblical Christian should be seeking out opportunities to exercise more responsibility in the kingdom of God rather than marshalling excuses to shun them.

In concentrating on what they have given up rather than on what they have received, they never lose the philosophical inclination to keep rewarding themselves.

3. Tithe and give with integrity.

This principle is easily misunderstood. It implies that every Christian should give, for that is a teaching of Scripture. However, it does not tell any individual how much he or she should be giving. The reason I suggest tithing and giving "with integrity" is because one's promise to give is made to God, not to a church or a cause. As such, the giver is responsible only to God. But God demands that our promises to Him be kept (Ecclesiastes 5:4-5).

When giving is a regular part of our financial management, and when it is done with integrity, great blessings result. This is not to say that we buy our way into God's favor so that He guarantees financial success. What it does say is that when we give first, when we do not hedge, but give from our full income, God honors the priority that we place on the financial needs of His kingdom by giving us wisdom to manage wisely whatever remains.

In Malachi 3:10, God actually encourages us to put Him to the test and promises blessings as we do so: "Bring the whole tithe into the storehouse, that there may be food in my house. Test me in this," says the LORD Almighty, "and see if I will not throw open the floodgates of heaven and pour out so much blessing that you will not have room enough for it."

I think the Lord refers here not to riches, necessarily, but the satisfaction of knowing that we are doing things His way—giving out of love and thankfulness, as an act of worship, not as a heavy obligation. This, in itself, suffices for the blessing promised.

4. Adopt a stewardship lifestyle.

A student about to graduate and enter residency asked me for financial counsel because he was overwhelmed with the student loans he had acquired. In analyzing his borrowing I discovered that he had bought a very expensive car, spending easily fifteen thousand dollars more than he might have for a new, well-equipped, reliable, lower-scale model. I asked him why he had bought that particular car. He replied, "The salesman reminded me that I had worked hard and had denied myself an awful lot. I figured I owed it to myself, so I went with what turned me on."

As Christians take seriously their stewardship of God's creation, they will become leaders in conserving scarce resources in order to serve future generations.

This reasoning, obviously not biblical, points out a subtle snare that can rob us of financial security and close many other options. The trap is buying what we don't need for all the wrong reasons, and going into debt to do so. I hear older practitioners, long past their training days, still recounting the hardships and privations of four years of dental school and a year or two of residency. In concentrating on what they have given up rather than on what they have received—the training and the benefits of a wonderful serving profession that allows us to do well by doing good—they never lose the philosophical inclination to keep rewarding themselves. They justify their actions as "delayed or postponed gratification," which can lead to a compulsive life-styles, distorted priorities and debt.

Christian professionals can be leaders in the movement to consume less, to buy necessities carefully and thoughtfully and to purchase luxuries with great care. Too often, impulse rules our buying decisions with neither comparison shopping nor any kind of long-range goals in mind. Some methods of controlling such impulses include the following:

"Dishonest money dwindles away, but he who gathers money little by little makes it grow" (Proverbs 13:11).

- Never go into debt to buy a luxury item or a "want," especially one that will be consumed before it is paid for.
- Allow a cooling-off period before finally deciding to buy. For a large item, two weeks to a month is an appropriate time to delay purchases. In many cases the item will have lost its allure.

• Buy only what you can buy with cash. "Saving up" is okay.

• Never pay interest on a credit card. Pay the balance in full every month.

• Resist the great American pastime of "going shopping." Play tennis or work out instead. The marketing of luxuries is a highly developed art that will press you to buy what you do not need, even against your better judgment. Very few of us can resist.

Those who remain debt-free, who have saved and increased their savings little by little, will have achieved financial security for their futures.

You will notice that these measures discourage borrowing to buy and consume, because incurring that kind of debt results in the most severe limitations on one of the most useful, satisfying, and blessed aspects of the Christian life, namely, serving God by serving others.

As Christians take seriously their stewardship of God's creation, they will become leaders in conserving scarce resources in order to serve future generations. They will use things all the way up, prevent the fouling of our environment, avoid waste such as carelessly discarded food, and they will recycle reusable resources.

5. Spend less than you earn.

You might be inclined to laugh at this point. Yet, in spite of the fact that it is so obvious, it is often ignored, especially by people with higher-than-average incomes.

Several aspects of this point are essential in order to understand and implement it. The first is that something should be done with the money which is not spent, which I will discuss at some length later in this chapter. That money should be used to take advantage of the "miracle" of compounded interest. Compounding interest for a long time is not only financially astute, but in line with a principle of Scripture (Proverbs 13:11).

Here's an easy example of the miracle of compounding interest: Say you save $265.80 per month at 12.5 percent interest for forty years, a reasonable career span from twenty-five to sixty-five years of age. Compounding of interest would grow the total of $127,584 saved over the years to $3,641,550 (without tax considerations). This type of compounding could develop in a tax-deferred retirement account such as an IRA or Keogh plan invested in a well-managed growth mutual fund.

But compounding of interest can work against us as well as for us. Borrowing on a credit card and making the minimum monthly payment, as many do, provides the *bank or credit-card company* with the kinds of returns mentioned above, and they have to put very little money at risk. No wonder the Bible says, "The borrower is servant to the lender" (Proverbs 22:7).

On the other hand, those who remain debt-free, who have saved and increased their savings little by little, will have achieved financial security for their futures. They can use the resources they have developed to increase their giving and to serve freely, especially when family responsibilities have diminished and their children have become self-sufficient.

Priorities ensure that essential obligations are met first; desires come after needs.

How to Live Debt-Free

If debt is so confining, if it limits options for a carefree, service-oriented present and future, what is the secret to living debt-free? A professional colleague asked me to speak at a conference he was arranging for a group of Christian health professionals in his community. "I attended one of your seminars and used your study guide for devotions with my wife," he said. "We are living debt-free for the first time in our lives. We can't get over the burden that has rolled off our shoulders. We are free to serve the Lord and finance our own teaching ministries in the Third World. What a blessing we are experiencing! We want to share it with others."

This is not an isolated incident. This particular colleague told me that he and his wife had never considered the possibility of paying off loans. They just kept plodding through the monthly payments and kept on borrowing with their credit card. Our society is so debt-oriented that no one had told this young family that an early goal for them should be debt-free living. Following are several steps that will help you take charge of your financial situation so that you are proactive and in control:

1. Set financial goals.

Without targets you will achieve nothing. Short-term goals of one or two years might include the elimination of all credit-card debt, saving a certain amount based on present or future educational needs for your children, and the establishment of a spending plan to help organize and apportion income and expenses. Long-term goals might include the funding of pension plans and IRAs, the purchase of a new automobile, the preparation of a will and estate plan with a charitable remainder trust, organization of giving through a private foundation, development of a business interest and inquiries into missions service, either foreign or domestic.

If giving is the highest priority in our spending plan, we will normally be able to keep our promises.

Once you've established goals, you can identity objectives to help reach them in an organized, measurable manner. Objectives are like signposts or checkpoints along the route of a marathon, for they break the task into achievable segments. As we achieve each objective, we build confidence that makes the next objective more easily attainable.

2. Develop a spending plan.

A spending plan organizes the family's finances so expenditures do not exceed income. Priorities ensure that essential obligations are met first; desires come after needs. Living according to priorities and with a spending plan, one realizes quickly whether sufficient income is present to support a particular lifestyle. If lifestyle outstrips income, major downsizing adjustments must be made. The reward of making these adjustments is financial freedom.

Most of the Christian financial management books found in a Christian bookstore have forms that you may use to develop such a plan. One of the most important steps is to list your expenditures in the order of your priorities. Here is a workable sample:

1. Giving;
2. Taxes;
3. Payment of loans, interest and principal;
4. Living expenses: housing, food, automobiles,

insurance, recreation, etc.;

5. Savings.

This list demands some explanation. Why, you may ask, is giving at the top of the list? Because I believe that when Christian do this, the habit of giving "firstfruits" becomes routine for the family. I know of a group that promised to support a missionary family working in a foreign country. The missionary had to return home because the group sent no money for several months, and only erratically prior to that. The missionary could not feed his children. When asked why the group had not kept its promise, the group's leader said, "Well, at the end of the month there was no money left. How could we meet our pledge?" This is not Christian giving. If giving is the highest priority in our spending plan, we will normally be able to keep our promises.

Borrowing must be taken seriously and should be considered with prayer and spiritual counsel, under the guidance of the Holy Spirit.

Second, taxes must be paid or one will languish in prison, unable to earn. And debts must be paid for the same reasons. But here, you must be careful to repay principal as well as interest, otherwise you'll never realize the freedom you're striving for. If you are deeply in debt, financial managers will often recommend that you make extra payments on high-interest loans in order to repay them as quickly as possible.

Many individuals, especially those raised in immigrant families where saving was a high priority, would place savings fourth on the list, and then live on what was left. If one's long-term goals were to fully fund IRAs and retirement plans, it would make sense to limit lifestyles in order to achieve such laudable goals. This is not easy for many families.

Living expenses should be allocated according to a workable formula which can be derived by using the charts in a financial planning book. If you're spending too much on housing or automobile payments or clothing, lifestyles adjustment must be made. Keeping in mind the reward—good provision for the family, orderly finances and a future free from obsession with financial problems—will provide powerful motivation to endure difficult adjustments until new behavior patterns become habitual.

Discipline will be necessary. You will be tempted to deviate from the plan. A Bible school professor once said, "First the testimony; then the test." Once you've decided to pursue a debt-free lifestyle, it will never be harder. As with the establishment of any budget, shopping list, or financial plan, impulse or point-of-purchase buying becomes a trap. One will have to do without, as strange as that may sound in our debt-tolerant society. The plan will only be as sound as the discipline exerted to adhere to it.

3. Control the credit card.

Because debt can destroy ministry or preempt opportunities to serve, Christians should try to live debt-free as soon as they can.

In order to adhere to a financial plan, you must control spending, not be controlled by it. You should do all shopping with a list and a resolve to not succumb to extras. Furthermore, the person in your family with the most self-control should do the shopping. Credit cards have become even more dangerous as it's become easy to use them at grocery stores. It's just too convenient to overspend. The bottom line is, if you can't control credit-card spending, you'll have to destroy the card and replace it with a debit card, which deducts the amount of purchase directly (and speedily) from your checking account.

Thoughts on Borrowing

Borrowing money is a spiritual matter. All material resources belong to God, and borrowing involves the use of material resources. Borrowing must be taken seriously and should be considered with prayer and spiritual counsel, under the guidance of the Holy Spirit. Here are some recommendations:

- Borrow money only with serious deliberation and full understanding and agreement between husband and wife.
- Never borrow for spending on consumable goods.
- Never borrow on a credit card. Credit card interest rates are the highest charged and, in some cases, are usurious.

Borrowing should never be predicated on whether or not you can make the monthly payments. In many cases credit-card repayment is structured so that the monthly payment does not include all the interest charged that month, so as to charge interest on accumulating interest, enriching only the credit-card lender. You should have a clear understanding of the devastating effects of compound interest working against you.

On the other hand:

Giving is a discipline that brings much blessing, joy and spiritual fruit.

    • Borrowing to buy a home in which the value of the house is more than the total borrowed (if, in other words, the loan is secured by the value of the house) generally makes sense, especially in a rising real-estate market. But even in this instance, if the real-estate market is deteriorating, the down payment should more than cover any potential deficiency between the sale price and the mortgage, should the house have to be sold.

    • Borrowing to set up a practice or for a business venture is also sensible if good value is received. However, one must be on guard against the recent practice of banks to have each partner in a venture personally guarantee the full value of the loan against his or her own personal financial assets. If the real-estate venture loses value greater than the amounts borrowed, the bank can and will seek full satisfaction for the "deficiencies" from each partner's personal holdings. This exposure can completely upset the financial plans of the unsuspecting.

How to Get Out of Debt

An aphorism that is trite but all too true is that it is easy to get into debt but very difficult to get out, especially when one does not realize the seriousness of the constraints that debt places on a family or individual. A health professional, knowing of my interest in the educational loan issue as it affects recruitment of missionaries, told me that repaying her student loans had interfered with her spiritual practices. "I have been in practice for ten years and am still paying off my educational loans. I haven't been able to tithe or go on short-term missions adventures. I will be glad when this debt is repaid!"

Our further conversations uncovered the following aspects of this debt millstone: the doctor had never considered anything but making the monthly payments on her loans; her husband was still indulging his pent-up delayed gratification from ten years previous; she was actually much deeper in debt than she had been upon entering practice, even though her student loans had been somewhat paid; the couple was unwilling to restrain their ever-expanding life-style in order to pay the loans as quickly as possible in order to be free to tithe and serve.

In 2 Corinthians 9 Paul makes it clear that our giving ought to be not only generous, but also cheerful.

Because debt can destroy ministry or preempt opportunities to serve, because payment of interest keeps one in servitude to the lender, and because we should be in servitude to God alone, I and many others have concluded that Christians should try to live debt-free as soon as they can. The more we learn to "want what we have," the freer we will be to seize the limitless opportunities to make disciples of all nations.

As a rule, high-interest consumer debt (credit-card companies and cards of retailers) should be paid off as soon as possible, and giving up excessive lifestyles and wants in order to do this are sensible sacrifices to achieve the goal. Then, remaining loans should be repaid in a systematic way until they are repaid in advance of the scheduled repayments. Exceptions might be, for example, an automobile loan at 2.8 percent interest made on an incentive program where the loan is secured by the value of the auto and one is earning more in interest in a certificate of deposit than the interest being charged on the loan.

If you cannot repay your loans on current terms, write or visit the lender and ask for more favorable terms. A sincere attempt to repay will often be met with a more manageable repayment plan. Some lenders may even extend a grace period so you can repay other loans with debilitating interest rates first. Note, however: Consolidation loans can be dangerous. Agree to these only if the repayment schedule allows for a reasonable interest rate and prepayment of principal without penalty.

Giving

I have alluded to giving several times in this chapter. It is such an important part of the faith disciplines of the Christian life that I would like to make several points regarding it. First, I know from longtime experience that giving is a discipline that brings much blessing, joy and spiritual fruit. I was fortunate; I was brought up in a family that practiced giving as a high priority, and I developed the giving habit early in life. Therefore it is difficult for me to be objective about giving. But experience—and the Bible—don't lie: "God loves a cheerful giver" (2 Corinthians 9:7).

That leads to my second point: Scripture clearly and firmly describes financial guidelines for the believer. All of us must study the kinds of giving described in the Bible and decide for ourselves what is appropriate in our own lives. Frankly, this issue is really between us and the Lord. Christ knows our hearts and sees our performance. We are answerable to Him. The amount of teaching devoted to this topic confirms that it is important to Him.

Develop the habit of writing your tithe check as the first payment made for the pay period.

The four types of tithing described below allow flexibility and different levels of growth as we mature in our faith. At various times many of us have used all of these, and sometimes combinations of two or more of them.

1. Storehouse Tithing (Malachi 3:9-12)

This teaching involves bringing the tithe to the storehouse, God's house, in order to support the temple, the priests and to care for the poor. Most interpret the amount of tithe to be at least 10 percent, or as much as 38 percent based on the Law.

Many believers conclude that the temple for us is represented by the local church and that our tithe should be given there. Support for parachurch ministries should come from anything given after the tithe. Many Christians argue about tithing, stating that it is outdated because it is based on the Law. But I have never met anyone who adhered to this method of giving, putting God to the test, who had not experienced the blessing promised in verse ten. Furthermore, we must be careful that, having objected to the legalism of this passage, we respond appropriately to the grace and freedom which are the spirit of giving in the New Testament.[1]

2. Proportional Giving (Acts 11:29)

In response to the physical needs of fellow Christians in a time of famine, "The disciples, each according to his ability, decided to provide help." The implication is that those who had more gave more, maybe more than a "legalistic" 10 percent.

3. Generous, Cheerful Giving (2 Corinthians 8:2-3; 9:6-8)

The Macedonian believers gave to their fellows in Jerusalem even though they were enduring severe trials and extreme poverty themselves. Their giving "overflowed with joy" and "welled up in rich generosity." This implies that the Macedonians gave more than 10 percent of what must have been a very meager income.

In 2 Corinthians 9 Paul makes it clear that our giving ought to be not only generous, but also cheerful. This is the demonstration of grace that God develops in us, grace that gives substance, meaning and fruitfulness to our good works.

There is a warning against giving reluctantly, grudgingly or out of a sense of duty. When our financial house is in order, when we are not beset by problems of debt and mismanagement, it is much easier to give out of a sense of blessing and with great joy—yet another reason to strive for debt-free living.

4. Faith-Promise Giving (2 Corinthians 8:3)

This form of giving started in the independent missions movement to support foreign missionaries. The verse in 2 Corinthians 8 describes the Macedonian Christians as having given "even beyond their ability." In Faith-Promise giving a person promises to give more to God than previously, not knowing where the funds will come from, but trusting the Lord to supply that which has been promised.

Don't postpone giving to a time in the future when you think you will be able to afford it. That time will likely never come.

Many people, including me, can testify to God's marvelous provision when we have promised to give by faith.

Guidelines for Giving

The following guidelines have helped me establish a routine for giving. I review them when I find myself feeling indifferent, irritated or distracted about sharing my financial rewards freely:

1. Give yourself first. Follow the example of the Macedonian believers who did this very thing (2 Corinthians 8:5). Be willing to stay and use your spiritual gifts and your training to grow the local church and help bring it to maturity. Be willing to go to use your profession to relieve physical needs and as a vehicle for introducing people to the love of Christ.

2. Give and tithe according to your own agreement with God. In order to be responsible and accurate in determining the amount you decide to give, keep—and review often—good records. Carefully kept records are a key to maintaining accountability before God and they allow us to easily adjust our current situation when we have more or less than anticipated income. As well, we ought to take full advantage of the tax laws as they encourage charitable activities by private institutions in order to spare government of further involvement in addressing human needs. Good records are also essential to verify tax deductibility.

Good stewardship brings a special responsibility to prepare for the future.

3. Tithe first and tithe the whole. Develop the habit of writing your tithe check as the first payment made for the pay period. Tithe on before-tax income. Praise God as you write the check. Pray that it will be used to bring others to a saving knowledge of our Lord Jesus Christ, and you will write the check with joy. It will also be easier to live on what remains as time goes on.

4. Begin tithing as early as possible. It is easier to start when income is low and increase as income increases. It is almost impossible to start at a high point, since it seems as though one is "giving up too much," and the lifestyle adjustments are too radical.

Don't postpone giving to a time in the future when you think you will be able to afford it. That time will likely never come.

At a conference, one of my fellow speakers asked if my wife and I would meet with her and her husband. We met in a private place. They wanted to talk about tithing, and told us that they had never been able to give . . . at all! They asked for encouragement and suggestions in how to get started. This mature family had substantial income from practice, book royalties and speaking engagements. I told them that we would stand with them and pray for them as they experienced the difficulty of getting started. When I suggested that they start small—by determining to give one percent of their income in the coming year—they looked at each other, shook their heads sadly and the conversation abruptly ended. I, too, was saddened—to see that they would miss the blessing of sharing their financial resources.

5. *Be involved in your giving.* Ministry and charitable organizations should be investigated and held accountable. Much money is wasted by "Christian" organizations with massive administrations and upscale salaries and lifestyle. Be faithful to the local church where you and your family are spiritually nourished. Follow your gifts with prayer. Look for new opportunities to increase your range of giving as God brings new people and organizations within your notice. Support start-up ministries within your sphere of interest and influence, especially if they are meeting needs that are being met in no other way.

These principles can also be applied to the lives of our families. We can begin by taking the time to include our children in pertinent discussions about family finances and financial planning.

6. *Aim to increase the percentage of your giving gradually.* As your family grows and children leave the nest you may be able to increase the amount you give. I know Christian professionals who share 50 to 70 percent of their incomes, though they have had to give up many extras to do so.

7. *Never use tithes as a weapon or bargaining chip.* From time to time we hear of a person who threatened to stop giving to the church if something was not done the way he or she desired. We must not follow our gifts with caveats, conditions and subtle messages. We should simply pray that God would give those who administer the gift wisdom and a keen sense of stewardship.

8. Keep balance in your giving. Give to the church. Give to a congregation in the Third World. Give to members of our profession who desire to serve God in difficult places and are held back by lack of support or the burden of student loans. Give to ministries fighting many battles in the inner cities of our nation, and keep a reserve in order to have God's money in hand when a crisis strikes.

Preparing for the Future

All of life is preparation for the next event, and good stewardship brings a special responsibility to prepare for the future. As we take seriously the present managerial role in which God has placed each one of us, we need to be ready for the widening role He has promised in Matthew 25:21:

> "Well done, good and faithful servant! You have been faithful with a few things; I will put you in charge of many things. Come and share your master's happiness!"

When we have kept our financial houses in order we will have prepared for a future that is free from worry about financial matters, allowing us to engage in ministry responsibilities that are even wider ranging and more fruitful than when we were active in practice. What a worthy goal.

Part of wise planning includes fully funding retirement plans in order to take advantage of the government's incentives to invest tax-deferred accounts with before-tax dollars. Making arrangements for retirement is neither an expression of greed nor a desire for a full barn in order to "take our ease, eat, drink and be merry." It is a way of providing for a future of ministry without having to be salaried or even reimbursed for expenses. It is a way to continue to increase giving so that our gifts will be used to encourage other dentists in their service to God. Students can be sponsored for short-term missions. Young dentists eager to serve God as career missionaries can be enabled to do so through programs such as Project MedSend.[2]

Careful financial planning can also have ministry implications as we learn more about opportunities such as Gift Annuities that give us income while it is needed, then revert to the designated Christian charity upon death. And astute—even shrewd—estate planning will radically reduce estate taxes so that we can provide our surviving spouse and heirs with increased income and our charitable favorites with generous bequests. Using Charitable Remainder Trusts, Revocable Trusts and Unitrusts will keep us giving long after we have been united with our Savior in Glory.

Applying Principles: Work and Home

This chapter does not purport to be a treatise on practice management, but the principles espoused here can be applied to the management of our practices to good effect. Practices run with good financial controls, with integrity in recording income and integrity with patients and staff, will flourish, especially if the functions of the practice are committed to God in prayer on a regular basis.

These principles can also be applied to the lives of our families. We can begin by taking the time to include our children in pertinent discussions about family finances and financial planning. We should also take their judgments into consideration when they reach certain levels of maturity.

Children learn easily to conserve resources, but they must be taught by words and example. Children can learn not to demand material things if they are taught that it is okay to be different from the world around them and they also understand that being different is a matter of our relationship with God.

Children ought to know about the struggles

involved in providing money for the family to live on. Occasionally they ought to see their parents at work. They need to have opportunities to earn money for themselves so that they learn the principles of managing money. Children can be taught to "save up" for some item that they desire, and as they grow older they can manage a yearly budget for clothing, for example, so that their desires are satisfied by the decisions they have made for themselves.

How blessed it is to be a follower of Jesus Christ. He, the Creator of the universe, cares about all aspects of our lives, and He has given us stewardship over a portion of that creation. May He give us wisdom to manage wisely.

Notes

1. CMDA does not have an official position on whether tithing is the New Testament standard for giving for Christians. However, all would agree that for the Christian, giving should be regular, proportional, cheerful and generous. Most Christian financial experts suggest that in America, where God has blessed us so generously, 10 percent may be less than proportional and generous for most.

2. Project MedSend, which repays educational loans for health professionals, allowing them to serve in missions without delay for debt repayment, can be reached at: Project MedSend, P.O. Box 1098, Orange, CT 06477-7098; Phone/Fax: (203) 891-8223; E-mail: medsend@juno.com; Web site: http://www.medsend.org.

Suggested Reading

Blue, Ron. *Master Your Money*. Nashville, TN: Thomas Nelson, 1986.

Blue, Ron. *The Debt Squeeze*. Pomona, CA: Focus on the Family, 1989.

Burkett, Larry. *Your Finances in Changing Times*. San Bernardino, CA: Campus Crusade for Christ, I975.

Burkett, Larry. *Debt-Free Living.* Chicago, IL: Moody Press, 1989.

Burkett, Larry. *The Complete Financial Guide for Young Couples.*Wheaton, IL: Victor Books, 1989.

Burkett, Larry. *The Coming Economic Earthquake.* Chicago, IL: Moody Press, 1990.

Burkett, Larry. *Using Your Money Wisely.* Chicago, IL: Moody Press, 1985.

Crosson, Russ. *Money and Your Marriage.* Dallas, TX: Word, 1989.

Friesen, Garry. *Decision Making and the Will of God* Portland, OR: Multnomah Press, 1980.

Yancey, Philip. "Learning to Live with Money." *Christianity Today*, 14 December 1984.

CHAPTER TEN

An Invitation to Live for Christ

by David Stevens, M.D.

All of the contributors to this book, fellow dentists for the most part, are motivated by the fact of their devotion to God in Jesus Christ. Much of what we've written cannot be fully experienced, appreciated or applied without the spiritual insights that come with knowing Christ. Most of us crave satisfaction of our spiritual hunger. We often look in the wrong places to satisfy that hunger and become disillusioned and discouraged. The Scriptures clearly teach that spiritual things must be spiritually discerned, and that in our natural state we cannot have that spiritual discernment (1 Corinthians 2:14).

As I travel across the country speaking to audiences of dental and medical students and practitioners, I constantly encounter a deep hunger for meaning and significance. An interest in spirituality—a new openness to God and what He is doing in the world—seems to be appearing. For some, it's a curiosity; for others the search is intense.

God calls each of us to Him in different ways. Sometimes that call is clear and straightforward. Other

You sense there is something more. You know intuitively that Someone had to call matter into existence. Something can't come from nothing. There has to be a Creator. And if He can truly create something from nothing, He must be God. And with all that power, He must be worth knowing.

Like greyhounds chasing a mechanical rabbit, we find ourselves running in circles, faster and faster, trying to beat out our colleagues for the elusive prize of happiness and fulfillment.

times, it takes us a while to realize exactly how God is working in our lives. Many of us, in and out of the healthcare professions, are living the story of the Prodigal Son (see Luke 15). We believe that we can run away from our heavenly Father to follow our own passions and desires. We chase satisfaction through prestige, accomplishment, money and sexual pleasure, but find real fulfillment unattainable. Like greyhounds chasing a mechanical rabbit, we find ourselves running in circles, faster and faster, trying to beat out our colleagues for the elusive prize of happiness and fulfillment. But the rabbit always runs just a little faster than we can run . . . or if by chance we do catch it, we find it tasteless and unsatisfying. We suddenly stop one day and wonder why in the world we ever entered the race.

Some men and women seem to have been running from God all their lives. Others were good kids, obeyed their parents, became exceptional students, went to Sunday school and church and even participated in the youth group. They may have even made a commitment to God at one time. Then they left home, and God, behind. Like the Prodigal mentioned above, they tried the world's best—but found only husks and empty seed pods.

Perhaps your life has been far different from that of the Prodigal. Maybe you are more like one of that parable's servants around the house. You were exposed to Christianity as a child through your parents, local church, or a friend—but you never made a decision to accept Christ personally. Perhaps you were turned off by inconsistencies in the life of someone who professed to be a Christian. You saw through the facade to the hypocrisy. So you threw off a personal relationship with God like you would a shirt that had been stained. Someone had tarnished the name of Jesus, so you decided to have nothing to do with Him.

Perhaps you have traveled another road altogether. Maybe you have never really heard the gospel story. You have only seen Christianity as another religion among many religions. Perhaps you view it is a crutch for the weak or disabled. With your intelligence and drive, the last thing you need is a crutch. You have made it is this far on your own. If you grit your teeth, work hard, and push on, you expect to do just fine.

Just maybe, though, you suspect that hard work isn't its own reward. There's more to life than professional achievement and honors—isn't there? Deep down inside you know things aren't right. The things you know you should do, you often don't do. Many of your relationships with others are in disarray. Your habits and actions are not healthy for you, and what's worse, they damage others. You have climbed over too many people to get where you are.

You sense that there is something more. You know intuitively that Someone had to call matter into existence. Something can't come from nothing. There has to be a Creator. And if He can truly create something from nothing, He must be God. And with all that power, He must be worth knowing.

If there is a God, is there some way you can know Him? Can He reveal Himself to you? Why did He create humanity in the first place, and give us souls? What's more, why did He create *you*—with your personality, skills and intellect? Could He have some purpose for your life?

These are tough questions worthy of careful examination. I challenge you to seek God. He is there, and He has a purpose for your life. More important, He wants a relationship with you—to become your friend. Hard to believe, isn't it? The God who called the universe into existence and created the intricacies of the human body loves and cares for *you*.

If there is a God, is there some way you can know Him? Can He can reveal Himself to you?

This is a fact recorded in the Scriptures and in history, as demonstrated in the lives of those who have sought Him. God has been involved in this world since He created it. He inspired the writing of the Bible so that everyone can know Him better. In His Word, the Bible, He tells us that sin entered the world when Adam and Eve turned their backs on Him and went their own way. Because of their choice, everyone is born into this world with sinful desires that lead to sinful actions. No matter how much we want to, we cannot live sinless lives. In the New Testament it says:

> "All have sinned and fall short of the glory of God. There is no one righteous, not even one" (Romans 3:23,10).

What this means is that we can't enter into a relationship with a holy God through our own goodness. We can't make ourselves good enough for God by deciding to act better and do nice things. Our spiritual genetics won't allow it. We're not capable. That is why God sent His Son, Jesus, into the world:

> "This is love: not that we loved God, but that he loved us and sent his Son as an atoning sacrifice for our sins" (1 John 4:10).

If you're ready to exchange emptiness for fullness, struggle for submission, I've got good news for you. Your heavenly Father wants you to come home.

Jesus' purpose in coming to earth was to pay the penalty for sin, which is death—spiritual death that comes from separation from God for eternity. When He died on the cross, He did so willingly, taking upon Himself the sins of all who would believe in Him—as if He were guilty Himself, though He had never sinned. He died in the place of all who would trust in Him.

Therefore, coming to God, starting a relationship with Him, is this simple: All you need do is ask for forgiveness and accept Jesus as your Savior. The moment that happens, though you may not feel it, everything changes. Not only are your sins forgiven, but God gives you a new life and fills that empty hole in your soul. Each of us writing this book has done this, and we can't recommend it strongly enough.

If you're ready to exchange emptiness for fullness, struggle for submission, I've got good news for you. Your heavenly Father wants you to come home. He has the door wide open and a feast is prepared! Friend, there are no husks and seed pods here. This meal will bring peace into your heart and joy into your soul.

Like the Prodigal, you just need to confess, as you would to a close friend, that you were wrong, that only Jesus can help you. Here is a prayer you may want to use as a model:

> "Dear God, I admit that I am a sinner and I understand that my sin separates me from You. I believe that Your Son, Jesus, being sinless, paid the penalty for all my sins when He died on the cross. I now receive Him as my Savior. Thank You for loving me and forgiving me and for giving me the gift of eternal life. Amen."

If we confess our sins, God promises in the Bible:

> "He is faithful and just and will forgive us our sins and purify us from all unrighteousness" (1 John 1:9).

When you make this decision and confession, many marvelous changes will occur in your life. You will possess every spiritual promise in the Scriptures—eternal life (John 3:16), spiritual discernment, freedom from guilt and the penalty of your sins and power to live a fulfilling life and to overcome life's battles. You will have a whole new family of believers in Christ, fellowship and relationships that are loving and vibrant, and new attitudes. The Holy Spirit of God, whom the Scriptures describe as one who walks alongside you to guide you, will teach you, encourage and fortify you. And . . . you will live in heaven with God forever when this life is over.

In summary, your decision places you, spiritually speaking, "in Christ," and the Bible says that anyone in Christ "is a new creation; the old has gone, the new has come" (2 Corinthians 5:17).

"For God so loved the world that he gave his one and only Son, that whoever believes in him shall not perish but have eternal life" (John 3:16).

If you need to know more before making this decision, I encourage you to read the Book of John in the New Testament. Or call us at the Christian Medical and Dental Associations (1-888-231-2637) and request a free copy of C. S. Lewis's book, *Mere Christianity*. It explains in much more detail who God is and what Jesus did for you and me.

If you have made that decision, you are now a brand-new person, like a newborn baby, in Christ. Just as an infant needs to grow and develop, so do you in your new faith. Let me give you some strategies that will help you grow into maturity in Christ, whether you have recommitted your life to Christ or have accepted Him for the first time as your Savior.

Strategies for Growth

1. Read the Bible daily.

Get a version that is understandable to you. The New International Version is an easy-to-understand

Entering dental school marks only the beginning of a lifelong study of dentistry. It is the same with your walk with Christ.

translation, as is *The Message*. Both are written in today's English. There are many other good Bibles available for study. Visit a local Christian bookstore to see all the options and ask for advice on which Bible to choose.

Then, find time to read a portion of the New Testament every day. God will reveal Himself to you through His Word. You may want to read right through the New Testament or read the Books of John and Romans first. The apostle Paul, author of several New Testament books, wrote, in his letter to Timothy:

> "All Scripture is God-breathed and is useful for teaching, rebuking, correcting and training in righteousness, so that the man of God may be thoroughly equipped for every good work" (2 Timothy 3:16-17).

2. Pray.

God wants you to get to know Him. A major way to do this is through prayer, just talking to Him as you would a friend. There is no special formula to use— just talk. Something I have found helpful in my own prayer life is a simple routine: I first praise God for who He is, then thank Him for the things He has done in my life and in the lives of others. Then I pray for others such as my family and friends. Finally, I pray for my own needs. The Bible lists many invitations to prayer, but one of the most specific is found in Philippians 4:6-7:

> "Do not be anxious about anything, but in everything, by prayer and petition, with thanksgiving, present your requests to God. And the peace of God, which transcends all understanding, will guard your hearts and your minds in Christ Jesus."

3. Find Christian friends for fellowship.

Fellowship is simply time spent with people ("fellows") of similar beliefs. Christian friends will help you grow in your faith and encourage you. You can find other believers through your local CMDA group, InterVarsity Christian Fellowship, Navigators, or Campus Crusade for Christ. Meet regularly with these friends to study the Bible together and pray.

4. Find a good church.

Attending church will help you become familiar with the Bible and God's ways, while also providing more Christian friends to help you grow. Ask your Christian friends for advice, then choose an evangelical church that teaches the truths of the Bible and worships in a style and format with which you are comfortable. If you find yourself in a church that does not emphasize the Bible's teachings, find another one. Why frequent a restaurant that doesn't serve real food?

5. Read good Christian books.

Many books are available to help new Christians in every area of life, from relationships to spiritual growth. Your local Christian bookstore is a good source for these, as are the many churches that have lending libraries. Pick books that deal with areas in which you have the greatest needs. CMDA is also a good source of a variety of types of books. Call: 1-888-231-2637 for more information.

6. Reach out to others.

Share your faith with your friends who don't know God yet. It will help you grow. Go on a domestic or overseas dental mission. CMDA's Global Health Outreach program will give you the opportunity to spend time with mature Christian dentists. They will teach you professionally, but more important, they will model what it means to be a Christian dentist.

In summary, entering dental school marks only the beginning of a lifelong study of dentistry. It is the same with your walk with Christ. It will be a fulfill-

"Therefore go and make disciples of all nations, baptizing them in the name of the Father and of the Son and of the Holy Spirit, and teaching them to obey everything I have commanded you. And surely I am with you always, to the very end of the age" *(Matthew 28:19-20).*

ing and thrilling journey as you grow in your faith and knowledge of God. You will find Him penetrating all that you do and becoming the pivot point around which your life rotates. Christ will become your source of joy and your reason for service. He will bring meaning to your life as He has to millions of others. Don't delay. Come to Jesus right now.

Contributors

Fred C. Bergamo, D.D.S., is a graduate of the University of Pennsylvania School of Dental Medicine. Dr. Bergamo is in general dental practice in Paramus, N.J., and has served as a Delegate and Trustee of the Christian Medical and Dental Associations. Together with Lew Bird, he coedited the book *A Personal Probe: Ethical Problems in Dental Practice.*

Lewis P. Bird, S.T.M., Ph.D., is Visiting Associate Professor of Christian Studies, Eastern College, St. Davids, Pa. He served as Eastern Regional Director of Christian Medical and Dental Associations for thirty-two years and was co-chair of the CMDA Ethics Commission.

J. Richard Bradbury, D.D.S., is a graduate of Ohio State University College of Dentistry, has served in the Public Health Service, and is now a full-time Associate Professor in the department of Restorative Dentistry, University of Maryland Dental School, where he is also adviser to the Student Christian Dental Association.

Kenneth B. Chapman, D.D.S., is a career missionary with Campus Crusade for Christ, working at Mengo Anglican Hospital in Kampala, the capital city of Uganda. There he heads the Dental Department, which is staffed by four dentists, two dental interns from the adjacent University Dental School and two public health dental assistants. Dr. Chapman has also served in Liberia and Korea; he's been in Uganda since 1979. He is a graduate of the University of Texas Dental Branch, Houston.

William C. Forbes, D.D.S., M.Div., is an Assistant Professor of Anatomy in the Biomedical Department of the University of Detroit Mercy School of Dentistry. Prior to assuming this position, he practiced general dentistry in Dover-Foxcroft, Maine, for 27 years. He is a graduate of Bangor Theological Seminary, and a licenced minister.

Peter C. McCutcheon, D.D.S., is a graduate of West Virginia Univ. School of Dentistry, currently serving in the Public Health Service in Alaska. He has been involved in mission projects in the Dominican Republic, Uganda and Eastern Russia.

Collin B. Sanford, D.M.D., is in the private practice of general dentistry in Avon, Conn. He is a graduate of the University of Connecticut School of Dental Medicine and is a part-time faculty member, teaching in the residency program as an associate clinical professor.

David Stevens, M.D., is Executive Director of the Christian Medical and Dental Associations. He has served as Director of World Medical Mission and as a medical missionary in Kenya for over a decade. Dr. Stevens is a graduate of Asbury College and the University of Louisville School of Medicine.

David Topazian, D.D.S., is President and CEO of Project MedSend, which repays educational loans for health professionals, allowing them to serve in missions without delay for debt repayment. A graduate of McGill University, he holds the M.Sc. in Pathology and the MBA in nonprofit management. Following many years in the practice of Oral & Maxillofacial Surgery and as a clinical professor at Yale University, he served with TEAM as a missionary in Venezuela for six and a half years. He is a past president of CMDA.

Richard G. Topazian, D.D.S., is Professor of Oral & Maxillofacial Surgery at the University of Connecticut School of Dental Medicine, and Director of Dental Services, Medical Ministry International. A graduate of McGill University, he has served as a missionary at the Christian Medical College and Hospital, Vellore, South India.